Training to Deliver Integrated Care

C. R. Macchi • Rodger Kessler
Editors

Training to Deliver Integrated Care

Skills Aimed at the Future of Healthcare

Springer

Editors
C. R. Macchi
Integrated Behavioral Health Programs
College of Health Solutions
Arizona State University
Phoenix, AZ, USA

Rodger Kessler
Integrated Behavioral Health Programs
College of Health Solutions
Arizona State University
Phoenix, AZ, USA

ISBN 978-3-030-07662-7 ISBN 978-3-319-78850-0 (eBook)
https://doi.org/10.1007/978-3-319-78850-0

This Springer imprint is published by the registered company Springer Nature Switzerland AG
The registered company address is: Gewerbestrasse 11, 6330 Cham, Switzerland

Preface

The emerging healthcare marketplace needs skilled behavioral healthcare practitioners (BHPs) and managers that prepare BHPs to be part of the medical team performing at the top of their training and credentials. Kathol, DeGruy, and Rollman (2014) note that the emerging primary care model requires behavioral clinicians specifically trained to work in new integrated care models. Multiple resources provide models and guidelines for integrated care delivery. In addition, there are disciplinary guidelines identifying skills for practitioners in specific disciplines (McDaniel et al., 2014). This book is not disciplinary. Rather it starts from the premise that defining integrated care defines the skill areas necessary to successfully practice in that setting, no matter your credential. We identify the instructional topics and processes to train the core skills and strategies needed by an integrated workforce.

This manual is relevant to the broadest array of training programs offered in varied settings (i.e., graduate degree training, certificate training, health system education, corporate workforce development). We refer to the reader of this manual as the trainer and the recipient of the training as the learner. Examples offered throughout the text apply to the learners within each setting. In addition, integrated behavioral practitioners may find this manual useful in considering and evaluating their own skills. Practitioners from multiple backgrounds perform varying degrees of behavioral healthcare service delivery. Throughout the text, we refer to the practitioner who is providing those services as the behavioral healthcare practitioner (BHP).

Section One

The first section describes emerging workforce development initiatives designed to support behavioral care in medicine. All practice and teaching are grounded in one's theory of what is needed. For our team, we are shaped by the American Academy of Family Physicians (AAFP) addendum to the Principles of the Patient Centered

Medical Home (PCMH) suggesting that the Medical Home is incomplete without the inclusion of behavioral health (Baird et al., 2014). We operate from a Three Worlds model of clinical care, noting the clinical, operational, and financial Worlds of Care simultaneously operate and must be understood and practiced (Peek, 2008). Our theory and language of integration is drawn from Peek's Lexicon of Collaborative Care (Peek & National Integration Academy Council, 2013). Last, we focus on the Triple Aim of healthcare – BHP's impacting on improved patient experience of care, improved clinical outcomes, and using evidence-supported care models to bend the overall healthcare cost curve. The above direct us to following dimensions of integrated care:

- *Evidence-based population healthcare*
  - An historic evidence base supports the effectiveness of behavioral interventions that are delivered by a variety of healthcare staff at the clinical, operational, and financial levels. Currently, much care delivery does not utilize this body of knowledge (Kathol et al., 2014).
- *Accomplish and measure Triple Aim outcomes*
  - Behavioral health and behavioral care are shaped by contemporary healthcare reform and design. The core focus of such redesign is care that reflects the Triple Aim objectives of calling for improved patient satisfaction with care, improved clinical outcomes, and reduced overall healthcare costs (Institute for Healthcare Improvement, 2015). Behavioral health has been sold on the premise that it is good, while contemporary healthcare transformation is focused on assessments based on metrics and measurements. We take the position that primary care integration has to be held to the same evaluation, measurement standards, and focus as the rest of healthcare.
- *"Move behavioral healthcare (BH) from carve out to carve in" as an integral part of comprehensive, integrated healthcare delivery*
  - The still prevalent "carve-out model" of financing healthcare separates medical and behavioral payment. There are no incentives or available financial supports to financially integrate systems. By implication, this separates care and de-incentivizes whole-person care. Without financial integration, improved behavioral management of medical issues and improved clinical outcomes and potential impact on overall healthcare costs are impossible. Mandates and movement toward whole-person care, Patient Centered Medical Homes (PCMHs), Accountable Care Organizations (ACOs), and bundled payments based on quality cannot occur without financial systems combining, with incentives for quality, whole-person care (Kessler, 2008).
- *Population health management (PHM) initiatives and programs*
  - The Affordable Care Act (Patient Protection and Affordable Care Act, 2010) generated a profound shift in care model. First, healthcare is primary care focused. Second, the focus of care shifts from individual patient to practice

panels with care delivered to the entire identified patient populations, primarily with multichronic disease morbidities (Pearson et al., 2005).
  - Effective, efficient, efficacious healthcare generates a focus on the business of healthcare management with the development, implementation, and evaluation of healthcare delivery all being driven by data, outcomes, and attention to efficiency cost and cost effect (Cummings & O'Donohue, 2008).

- *Healthcare delivery improvements and efficiencies*
  - Care delivery improvements and cost efficiencies can only be accomplished by approaches that employ applied, translational, continuous, quality improvement efforts that drive the planning and execution of integrated care. These efforts must assist model development, operational, and financial processes, and practice workflow issues that enable seamless integrated care that improve quality and office function without generating barriers such as increased staff work burdens, increasing time on tasks, or limiting provider staff and patient access (van Eeghen, Littenberg, Holman, & Kessler, 2015).

- *Measuring levels of integrated healthcare*
  - Model of care relates to the definitions of the varying levels of integrated care. For the first time, the Lexicon of Collaborative Care (AHRQ) identified the core dimensions of integration. In addition, over the last 3 years, the Practice Integration Profile (PIP) has operationalized the dimensions of the lexicon into a valid measure of integration dimensions and total integration scores that allow practices to target a desired degree of engagement at each dimension of integration (Macchi et al., 2016). Providing a reliable, valid measurement tool now allows the healthcare field to ask a critical question: "Do degrees of integration affect types and degrees of outcome?" (Kessler, 2015; Kessler et al., 2015)

- *Integrated healthcare workforce training*
  - From degree education to ongoing professional training, the workforce should match current and expected levels of system while tooling the workforce to make a transition to the next level of prepared integrated care workforce (McDaniel et al., 2014).

- *Evaluating integrated care effectiveness using the EHR*
  - This is the time of evaluating our efforts and assessing their outcomes. Evaluation models must be rapid, valid, and actionable (Kessler & Glasgow, 2011) to evaluate healthcare model development and care delivery at every stage. Currently, the RE-AIM framework greatly assists identification and measurement of core, on-the-ground issues including Reach, Effectiveness, Adoption, Implementation, and Maintenance (Glasgow, 2006).
  - The electronic health record (EHR) will be the source of patient identification, engagement, selection of clinician and strategy and measuring outcomes, and behavioral care needs (Table 1).

Table 1 Crosswalk of dimensions of integrated care with Three Worlds and Triple Aim

Dimensions of integrated care	Three Worlds dimensions (Clinical, operational, financial)	Triple Aim outcomes (Patient satisfaction, improved outcomes, impact on costs)
Evidence-based healthcare	C, O, F	PS, IO, C
Accomplish and measure triple aim outcomes	C, O, F	PS, IO, C
"Move behavioral health (BH) from carve out to carve in" as an integral part of comprehensive, integrated healthcare delivery	O, F	PS, IO, C
Population Health Management (PHM) initiatives and programs	C, O	PS, IO, C
Healthcare delivery improvements and efficiencies	O, F	PS, IO, C
Measuring levels of integrated healthcare	O	PS, IO, C
Integrated healthcare workforce training	C, O, F	PS, IO, C
Evaluating integrated care effectiveness using the EHR	C, O, F	PS, IO, C

Section Two

This section (Chaps. 2 and 3) reviews the state of the science related to medical and behavioral integration. Integrated practice models and core competencies are identified and broad guidelines are presented for designing, implementing, and evaluating an effective training plan. Chapter 2 reviews current integrated behavioral healthcare models with a focus on the conceptual frameworks that have been used to guide the development of those models that allow us to observe how each model is distinct and overlaps with the others. Chapter 3 identifies the interprofessional skills needed to provide behavioral health effectively in the primary care setting. As we focus on key training and workforce development issues, we add training as a fourth world (i.e., clinical, operational, financial, and training) (Peek, 2008). We focus on core competencies including the identification and use of performance metrics.

Section Three

This section (Chaps. 4, 5, 6, 7, 8, 9 and 10) focuses on the structure and content of an existing doctoral-level integrated behavioral health degree program. The chapters in this section reflect the core of the manual that addresses the pedagogical priorities for each training component. Each chapter describes instructional delivery methods for presenting key didactics through asynchronous, online delivery, and provide learner practice experiences that are supported through synchronous,

Table 2 Chapter overview grid

Chapter overview	
Domains	*Identifies the related dimensions of integration (listed above) that are addressed in the chapter*
Key points	*Specifies the key training implications related to the chapter topic*
Student learning objectives (SLOs)	*Identifies specific, measurable statements to focus training development and delivery that is designed to support learner engagement and outcomes*
Instructional strategies	*Reviews pedagogical approaches and instructional tools that effectively support learning*
Evaluating learning	*Explores performance metrics and measurement strategies to determine that a learner has gained the knowledge and effectively demonstrates related skills*

videoconferencing consultation. These delivery methods are designed to support increasing student accessibility to learning and application in diverse contexts. Each chapter provides information related to a specific topic along with sample questions for designing learning objectives and teaching tips for course delivery and evaluation of learner comprehension and application. The chapters are divided into several sections in a parallel layout that includes an identified topic, guiding instructional design questions, and specific examples reflecting ways to deliver the curriculum.

The trainer's primary task begins with assisting the learner in making the conceptual shift "from current to emerging healthcare practices." Each topic is described while identifying the development of a related set of skills and training implications. Suggestions for the design and delivery of instruction as well as the support and evaluation of the learner's skill development conclude each chapter. Table 2 serves as the framework that will appear at the beginning of each chapter summarizing the key training issues addressed in that chapter.

The contributors were asked to develop chapters that are organized under the following subsections:

1. Background
   - (i) Review of historical/traditional approaches to the topic and related training issues.
   - (ii) Description of the impact of key conceptual and operational shifts on patient outcomes and associated training approaches. Tables are provided that compare old versus new models.
   - (iii) Practitioner performance barriers to integration that suggest the need for focused training and support (provide a checklist of related barriers).
2. Learning objectives are designed to address changes at multiple levels.
3. Practitioner performance barriers to integration
   - (i) Suggest the need for focused training and support
   - (ii) Provide a checklist of related barriers

4. Training or skill acquisition – learner assignments
   (i) Development and performance of practitioner core competency skills
   (ii) Support of team-based care performance improvements
   (iii) Impact of behavioral health service provision on utilization, costs, and ROI
5. Measurement – evaluation/rubrics that
   (i) Measure the effects of training
   (ii) Specify measures and metrics for expected performance impact and outcomes
   (iii) Provide a template and examples for calculating impact and outcomes
6. Provide a template that invites the trainer to develop a case example from their learners' caseload that illustrates practical implications of shift toward increased integration. Focus this section on identification of the training priorities that are required to prepare the learners for effectively addressing the issue (examples from varying system levels – patient, provider, practice, health system, healthcare policies).

The chapters in Section 3 address the training objectives and strategies that support learner skill development in key areas involved with comprehensive integrated healthcare services. Each chapter provides guidelines for designing, implementing, and evaluating training objectives that are focused on those skills. Chapter 4 addresses the skills needed to design, develop, implement, and evaluate population-based programs that use population health management approaches to care. Chapter 5 covers quality improvement, research, and outcomes-informed skills that are involved with practice-based research. These skills support the development and transformation of healthcare delivery and related business models. Chapter 6 focuses on training that prepares BHPs to develop distinct and complementary roles and effectively perform with other providers on medical teams. Chapter 7 explores ways to develop healthcare management skills that are needed to recognize and address the connections among provider performance, patient outcomes, utilization rates, and healthcare costs. Chapter 8 focuses on training strategies supporting learner development of business entrepreneurship skills that are needed to connect integrated healthcare practice with the business of healthcare. This chapter also addresses the unique instructional strategies that support the development of business plans focused on carving out a niche in an evolving marketplace. Chapter 9 explores the key elements of effective internship, training, and workforce development programs that provide applied experiences designed to support learner skill development. This chapter addresses the employment of key performance metrics to determine that core competencies simultaneously engage the Three Worlds (clinical, operational, and financial) of healthcare delivery. Chapter 10 provides a unique training approach to statistics and program evaluation. The approach focuses on the principles, strategies, and techniques of applied research design and data analysis for clinical practitioners and healthcare managers.

Section Four

The final section (Chaps. 11 and 12) addresses current and future training and infrastructural support for integrated healthcare delivery programs and services and transformational systems change. Chapter 11 addresses training issues related to the creation of workforce development CEUs/CMEs programs. This chapter focuses on the development of interprofessional, integrated care training programs that facilitate system-level transformation. Chapter 12 addresses the ethical, legal, and professional issues that are unique to team-based integrated healthcare practice.

Phoenix, AZ, USA

C. R. Macchi
Rodger Kessler

References

Baird, M., Blount, A., Brungardt, S., Dickinson, P., Dietrich, A., Epperly, T., et al. (2014). Joint principles: Integrating behavioral health care into the patient-centered medical home. *Annals of Family Medicine, 12*(2), 183–185. https://doi.org/10.1370/afm.1633.

Cummings, N. A., & O'Donohue, W. T. (2008). Tailoring collabroative care to fit the need: Two contrasting case studies. In R. Kessler & D. Stafford (Eds.), *Collaborative medicine case studies: Evidence in practice*. New York, NY: Springer.

Glasgow, R. E. (2006). RE-AIMing research for application: Ways to improve evidence for family medicine. *Journal of the American Board of Family Medicine, 19*, 11–19.

Institute for Healthcare Improvement. (2015). IHI Triple Aim measures. Retrieved from http://www.ihi.org/engage/initiatives/TripleAim/Pages/MeasuresResults.aspx

Kathol, R. G., Degruy, F., & Rollman, B. L. (2014). Value-based financially sustainable behavioral health components in patient-centered medical homes. *Annals of Family Medicine, 12*(2), 172–175. https://doi.org/10.1370/afm.1619.

Kessler, R. (2008). Integration of care is about money too: The health and behavior codes as an element of a new financial paradigm. *Families, Systems, & Health, 26*(2), 207–216.

Kessler, R. (2015). Evaluating the process of mental health and primary care integration: The Vermont Integration Profile. *Family Medicine and Community Health, 3*(1), 63–65.

Kessler, R., & Glasgow, R. E. (2011). A proposal to speed translation of healthcare research into practice: Dramatic change is needed. *American Journal of Preventative Medicine, 40*(6), 637–644. https://doi.org/10.1016/j.amepre.2011.02.023.

Kessler, R., van Eeghan, C., Mullin, D., Auxier, A., Macchi, C. R., & Littenberg, B. (2015). Measuring behavioral health integration in primary care settings. *Health Psychologist*. https://div38healthpsychologist.com/2015/03/13/research-in-progress-measuring-behavioral-health-integration-in-primary-care-settings/

Macchi, C. R., Kessler, R., Auxier, A., Hitt, J., Mullin, D., van Eeghen, C., & Littenberg, B. (2016). Describing and measuring levels of integrated behavioral healthcare: Improving quality, improving research. *Families, Systems & Health, 34*(4), 334–341.

McDaniel, S. H., Grus, C. L., Cubic, B. A., Hunter, C. L., Kearney, L. K., Schuman, C. C. et al. (2014). Competencies for psychology practice in primary care. *American Psychologist, 69*(4), 409–429. https://doi.org/10.1037/a0036072.

Pearson, M., Wu, S., Schaefer, J., Bonomi, A., Shortell, S., Mendel, P. et al. (2005). Assessing the implementation of the chronic care model in quality improvement collaboratives. *Health Services Research, 40*(4), 978–996.

Peek, C. J. (2008). Planning care in the clinical, financial, and operational worlds. In R. Kessler & D. Stafford (Eds.), *Collaborative medicine case studies: Evidence in practice* (pp. 25–38). New York: Springer Science.

Peek, C. J., & National Integration Academy Council. (2013). *Lexicon for behavioral health and primary care integration: Concepts and definitions developed by expert concensus*. Rockville, MD: AHRQ Publication Retrieved from http://integrationacademy.ahrq.gov/sites/default/files/Lexicon.pdf.

van Eeghen, C., Littenberg, B., Holman, M., & Kessler, R. (2015). Integrating behavioral health in primary care using Lean Workflow Analysis: A quality improvement case study. *Submitted for publication*.

Contents

Section I Introduction

1 **Introduction** 3
Rodger Kessler and C. R. Macchi

Section II Overview of Integration: State of the Science

2 **Integrated Behavioral Healthcare Models** 15
Colleen Clemency Cordes, Jeff Reiter, and Lesley Manson

3 **Enhancing Team-Based Skills in Primary Care: A Competency-Based Approach to Training and Workforce Development** 37
C. R. Macchi and Rodger Kessler

Section III Training the Workforce for Integrated BH Care

4 **PHM-Focused Healthcare Delivery** 65
Sue Dahl-Popolizio and Stephanie Brennhofer

5 **Quality Improvement, Performance Management, and Outcomes: Lean Six Sigma for Integrated Behavioral Health** 79
Ronald O'Donnell and Rodger Kessler

6 **BHP Performance on Medical Teams** 103
Lesley Manson

7 **The Business Case for Integrated Behavioral Healthcare Delivery** 119
Ronald O'Donnell

8 Business Entrepreneurship: The Integrated Behavioral Health Business Plan 143
Ronald O'Donnell and Sue Dahl-Popolizio

9 Graduate Internship Training of Integrated Behavioral Health in Primary Care (IBHPC) 161
C. R. Macchi and Colleen Clemency Cordes

10 Applied Data Analysis and Evaluation 177
Felicia Trembath and Stephanie Brennhofer

Section IV Supporting System Changes for Integration

11 Workforce Development: Identifying Continuing Education Needs and Programs for Integrated Behavioral Health Training 207
Colleen Clemency Cordes

12 Ethical Integrated Healthcare 213
Lesley Manson

Index 225

List of Figures

Fig. 1.1 Levels of training objectives 8

Fig. 2.1 Stages of integrating a model of care. 26

Fig. 3.1 Dimensions of team-based care – roles, responsibilities, and participation. 39
Fig. 3.2 Example of layered competencies 39
Fig. 3.3 Dimensions of healthcare practice – clinical, operational, financial 41
Fig. 3.4 Training phases 46
Fig. 3.5 Linked program and course components 53

Fig. 4.1 Relationships among population health, PHM, and public health 68
Fig. 4.2 PHM patient identification and stratification steps 70
Fig. 4.3 Financial ROI 74
Fig. 4.4 Cost-saving ROI 74

Fig. 5.1 Value stream map for diabetes clinic patient visit 83
Fig. 5.2 Causes of waste in a patient office visit 85
Fig. 5.3 The PDSA cycle. 86

Fig. 6.1 Workforce training cycle 110

Fig. 7.1 Integrated behavioral health models, costs, and revenues 123

Fig. 10.1 The relationship of confounders 182
Fig. 10.2 The relationship of confounders: smoking example 183
Fig. 10.3 Decision tree for choosing a statistical test 187
Fig. 10.4 Normal distribution curve 192
Fig. 10.5 Types of skewness 193
Fig. 10.6 Types of kurtosis 193

List of Tables

Table 1	Crosswalk of dimensions of integrated care with Three Worlds and Triple Aim	viii
Table 2	Chapter overview grid	ix
Table 1.1	Example rubric of exposure outcomes	9
Table 1.2	Example rubric of skill development outcomes	10
Table 1.3	Example rubric of competency outcomes	10
Table 2.1	Strategies linked to models of integrated care	28
Table 3.1	Integrated team-based approach: common objectives, involvement, and outcomes	40
Table 3.2	Crosswalk of core competencies on three world dimensions	43
Table 3.3	Early phase training objectives: foundations of team development and team-based care	47
Table 3.4	The Five As model: a guide for a team-based approach	48
Table 3.5	Integrated team-based training development plan	50
Table 3.6	Example assignment assessment rubric	52
Table 4.1	Historical shifts in population health management education	67
Table 4.2	PHM development planning guide	73
Table 5.1	Quality measures by domains and subdomains by Behavioral Health and General Medical Groupings	89
Table 5.2	Quality targets of phase 1 VBP of the mental health integration program and corresponding fidelity measures	91
Table 5.3	Learning objectives	92
Table 5.4	Lean Six Sigma competencies, learning objectives and activities, and measurement	93
Table 6.1	IPE Competencies and training application	106
Table 6.2	Team-based resources	111

Table 6.3 Team-based skill and performance measurement and training priorities . . . 114
Table 6.4 Depression treatment team-based skill and performance training plan examples. . . . 117

Table 7.1 Comparison of competencies for clinical providers in primary care. . . . 125
Table 7.2 Domain 1: Competencies for calculating program costs. . . . 127
Table 7.3 Domain 2: Competencies for projecting revenue . . . 128
Table 7.4 Domain 3: Competencies for integrated behavioral health business case pro forma . . . 129
Table 7.5 Domain 4: Competencies for integrated behavioral health return on investment formula . . . 130

Table 8.1 Grading rubric for the behavioral health business plan written assignment. . . . 145
Table 8.2 Grading rubric for the behavioral health business plan pitch presentation. . . . 146

Table 9.1 Sample of BHP performance evaluation tool – conceptual and professional development domain . . . 169
Table 9.2 BHP performance metrics and targets. . . . 171
Table 9.3 Sample of BHP performance evaluation tool – practice management domain . . . 173
Table 9.4 Sample training and assessment planning template . . . 174

Table 10.1 Change in statistical use over time . . . 179
Table 10.2 Measurement scales. . . . 182
Table 10.3 How reality and the decision made can lead to a correct conclusion or error . . . 184
Table 10.4 Types of study designs. . . . 186
Table 10.5 Sample codebook . . . 189
Table 10.6 Parametric tests and the equivalent nonparametric tests . . . 194
Table 10.7 Sample evaluation template. . . . 196
Table 10.8 Sample training template. . . . 199

Table 12.1 Principles of ethical practice . . . 215
Table 12.2 Integrated ethical, legal, and professional decision-making chart . . . 217
Table 12.3 Integrated ethical, legal, and professional decision-making tool . . . 218
Table 12.4 Legal, ethical, and professional case topics. . . . 220
Table 12.5 Suggested applied assignments . . . 222

About the Authors

C. R. Macchi is currently with Arizona State University as a Clinical Associate Professor, Academic Program Lead for the programs in Integrated Behavioral Health, and Associate Chair of Internship Programs in the College of Health Solutions. He was trained as a systems therapist receiving his doctorate in family therapy from Kansas State University. He is a Licensed Marriage and Family Therapist in Arizona, an Approved Supervisor with the American Association of Marriage and Family Therapists (AAMFT), and a Certified Family Life Educator (CFLE) with the National Council on Family Relations (NCFR). For the past 6 years in the Doctor of Behavioral Health Program, he has led the development of the internship program to establish key learning objectives, institute student- and program-level performance metrics, train the faculty who support student interns to meet program goals and objectives, develop an intern assessment tool, and develop an online data management system to monitor student intern progress. He consulted with integrated healthcare field experts and developed an integrated behavioral health provider performance rubric that assesses doctoral student interns' development of core competencies. He also developed and teaches a course focused on training behavioral health providers to work effectively with couples and families in primary care.

Dr. Macchi is involved in several grant-funded research initiatives focused on the development, implementation, and evaluation of workforce development programs. The trainings have been offered in-person and online, synchronous and asynchronous, within graduate degree programs and as stand-alone continuing education programs. As a Principal Investigator, Dr. Macchi is leading a team that is developing an asynchronous, online training program designed for adult learners who are providers of integrated team-based healthcare in primary care settings. This initiative is funded by a 5-year Patient-Centered Outcomes Research Institute (PCORI) subcontract with the University of Vermont School of Medicine and in collaboration with a team from the University of Massachusetts Medical School. He is on a team overseeing the Arizona State University Screening, Brief Intervention, and Referral to Treatment (SBIRT) Training and Implementation Collaborative (ASU-STIC). This 3-year Substance Abuse and Mental Health Services Administration

(SAMHSA) grant-funded project works with five ASU degree programs (i.e., Nursing, Social Work, Clinical Psychology, Counseling Psychology, and Integrated Behavioral Health) focused on developing sustainable training programs for clinical students preparing to work in medical and mental health settings. He works with a research team that has developed and validated the Practice Integration Profile (PIP) that measures practice-level integration.

As a Co-Investigator on several previous Centers for Medicare and Medicaid Services (CMS)-funded grants, he led a research team that developed, implemented, and evaluated a multi-delivery training program (i.e., in-person, videoconferencing, and asynchronous online learning modules) designed to support clinicians' use of evidence-based family therapy practices. Dr. Macchi administered the projects in collaboration with other statewide stakeholders including the Department of Social and Rehabilitative Services of Kansas, the Association of Community Mental Health Center Directors, and Kansas Health Solutions (a state Medicaid-contracted organization). As the project manager for a 5-year, United States Department of Agriculture (USDA) grant-funded initiative, he collaborated with key stakeholders in three Kansas counties training teens to engage with and support their communities' efforts to increase physical activity.

He has authored peer-reviewed articles related to health behavior change and integrated healthcare measurement. He has presented at national conferences on additional topics related to educational training strategies and techniques.

Rodger Kessler is a Health Psychologist who practiced previously in Family Medicine for over 25 years. He is currently with Arizona State University as a Chair of Research and Evaluation with the programs in Integrated Behavioral Health and a Professor of Biomedical Informatics in the College of Health Solutions. He is Co-Principal Investigator on the Integrated Behavioral Health in Primary Care (IBH-PC) Comparative Effectiveness Trial supported through PCORI, to evaluate the outcomes of co-located and integrated models of behavioral care as part of primary care. He also leads a national expert team, funded by the Sunflower Foundation, to identify core clinical process and financial metrics for integrated care.

Dr. Kessler has designed, implemented, and evaluated the effectiveness of many integration projects in family medicine, internal medicine, OB-GYN, neurology, gastroenterology, surgery, and anesthesiology, as well as three integrated Vermont Fletcher Allen Health Care Patient-Centered Medical Home Integration Pilots. He was Principal Investigator of a SAMHSA-funded multi-department initiative training medical residents, nurses, and social work students in team-based integrated care.

In his research career, he is Director of the Collaborative Care Research Network (CCRN), a subnetwork of the National Research Network (NRN), and Senior Scientist of the American Academy of Family Physicians. He was Principal Investigator of an NIH research project to develop a toolkit to assist practices that implement behavioral health and health behavior care in primary care. He leads a national team of investigators that developed the *Practice Integration Profile*, an electronic practice level self-report identifying level of Primary Care Behavioral Health.

He has previously edited, *Collaborative Medicine Case Studies: Evidence in Practice* with Dale Stafford, MD, and the *Handbook of Clinical Health Psychology* with Christine and Chris Hunter, both published by Springer Publishers. He has over 50 other refereed publications.

Colleen Clemency Cordes is currently with Arizona State University as an Assistant Dean and on faculty with the programs in Integrated Behavioral Health in the College of Health Solutions. She is a licensed counseling psychologist. Her clinical background and training have almost exclusively been in traditional medical settings, having worked in primary care settings at Banner Good Samaritan Hospital in Phoenix, Arizona; the VA Hospital in Long Beach, California; the Edith Nourse Rogers Memorial Veterans Hospital in Bedford, Massachusetts; and HonorHealth's Neighborhood Outreach and Access to Health (NOAH) clinics. She received a certificate in Primary Care Behavioral Health from the University of Massachusetts Medical Center and completed didactic training programs in biofeedback and clinical hypnosis from the Cambridge Health Alliance, an affiliate of Harvard Medical School. She is currently on the board of directors for the Collaborative Family Healthcare Association (CFHA). Her research interests focus on primary care behavioral health and workforce development for integrated primary care. Dr. Clemency Cordes is also a proud Sun Devil, having graduated from the Counseling Psychology program at Arizona State University in 2009.

Jeff Reiter is currently with Arizona State University as a Clinical Associate Professor with the programs in Integrated Behavioral Health in the College of Health Solutions. He is coauthor (with Patricia Robinson, PhD) of one of the leading books on primary care integration, titled, *Behavioral Consultation and Primary Care: A Guide to Integrating Services*. The first edition was published in 2007 and the second in 2015. Currently, he works as a Subject Matter Expert with the Department of Defense, helping them implement integrated care on military bases around the world. Previously, starting in 2002, he developed and led large integrated primary care services in Seattle, first in community health and then in the commercial sector. Dr. Reiter is on the Board of the Collaborative Family Healthcare Association (CFHA), and in 2014, he and Chris Hunter, PhD, established within CFHA the first organized group dedicated to the Primary Care Behavioral Health (PCBH) model of integrated care. In 2016, CFHA honored Dr. Reiter with its first "Outstanding Contributions to the PCBH Model Award." In 2009, he and Mountainview Consulting Group, Inc., were awarded the American Psychological Association's "Presidential Award for Innovative Practice," for their work in integrating primary care. Dr. Reiter frequently speaks to, and consults with, organizations around the country on the topic of integrated primary care. He is interested in primary prevention, medically underserved populations, the behavior change process, primary care, and population health. Before working in integrated primary care, he spent 8 years as an active-duty psychologist in the US Air Force. He received his PhD in clinical psychology from the University of Vermont, and holds an ABPP in behavioral psychology.

Lesley Manson is currently with Arizona State University as a Clinical Assistant Professor and Assistant Chair of Integrated Initiatives with the programs in Integrated Behavioral Health in the College of Health Solutions. Further she provides consultation related to building and training for fiscally sustainable Integrated Care Behavioral Health programs. She has spent over a decade providing direct service. Her dedication to behavioral health and integrated care models led her to directing behavioral health programs, providing continuing education to healthcare providers, and developing workshops and trainings for behavioral health and primary care providers to be successful and integral members of healthcare teams. Her specialty is within the area of building fiscally sustainable integrated healthcare with identifiable return on investment and cost savings. She has advanced experience in continuous quality improvement, behavior change, and standardization and outcome measurement for behavioral health programs integrated into primary care. Dr. Manson has spearheaded multidisciplinary teams for primary care process improvement and population-specific quality improvement and standardization, which has led to improved healthcare outcomes, enhanced quality assurance, increased compliance and patient engagement, and reduced healthcare costs. She was an integral member of teams for the development of electronic medical health records with integrated shared behavioral health focusing on standardization, best practices, and evidence-based techniques.

Her history as a healthcare executive has led her to voluminous national presentations on integration with both clinical and management focus and providing consultation and training for primary care and medical/behavioral organizations in developing and auditing for integrated care quality and fiscal sustainability. She develops train-the-trainer and additional educational programming for numerous contracted agencies such as Centers for Medicare and Medicaid, National Center for Interprofessional Practice and Education, and various federal and independent medical associations and organizations.

Historically, she has been an active member of her local and national professional primary care and behavioral health organizations, serving on numerous boards, receiving recognitions, and was former president of the North Coast Association of Mental Health Professionals in California and has co-chaired the PCBH and pediatric special interest groups for the Collaborative Family Healthcare Association. She was honored with certificate training from Johnson & Johnson UCLA Health Care Executive Program. She is also a master trainer for the Institute for Healthcare Communication and conducts workshops in the area of clinician-patient interaction, team-based care, and communication to meet healthcare's triple/quadruple aim. She has numerous publications on integration and is a coauthor of *Integrating Behavioral Health into the Medical Home*.

Sue Dahl-Popolizio is currently with Arizona State University as a Clinical Assistant Professor with the programs in Integrated Behavioral Health in the College of Health Solutions. She is an occupational therapist and certified hand therapist, and she holds a doctorate in behavioral health from ASU. She has over 20 years of experience in multiple medical settings providing occupational therapy (OT) services for patients with issues ranging from minor medical and behavioral health issues to trauma. Her current work and research/publication foci include population health management in integrated primary care, and the role of OT on the integrated interprofessional primary care team, especially as related to chronic conditions.

Stephanie Brennhofer is currently with Arizona State University as a Research and Evaluation Specialist with the programs in Integrated Behavioral Health in the College of Health Solutions. She was clinically trained as a registered dietitian nutritionist receiving her Master of Science degree in Nutrition from Arizona State University. She also holds a Master of Public Health degree in Applied Epidemiology from the University of Arizona. Stephanie is a public health researcher and has been involved in various research projects since 2010. Her predominant contributions to research studies have been in methodological design and statistical analyses. Primarily, her research has focused on the social determinants of health, underserved populations, and infectious diseases. She has published her findings in peer-reviewed journals and has presented nationally. Stephanie lectures undergraduate and graduate students in public health and integrated health care on study design, methodology, and statistical analyses.

Ronald O'Donnell is currently with Arizona State University as a Clinical Professor and International Partnership Program Manager with the programs in Integrated Behavioral Health in the College of Health Solutions. Dr. O'Donnell is a psychologist and founding Director of the Doctor of Behavioral Health program (2008–2014) in the College of Health Solutions. He is President of SunCrane Health Solutions, LLC, an international behavioral health consulting company, and is Education Director for HSAIG, a medical consultation and training company.
Dr. O'Donnell is a leader in the field of education and training on "integrated behavioral healthcare," the use of behavioral interventions to improve both medical and psychiatric problems, such as diabetes and depression. He led the effort to establish the Doctor of Behavioral Health program and has continued to contribute to the ongoing development of the curriculum, internship training, and expansion to include both clinical and health management concentrations. He is now working on the development of international education programs for the College of Health Solutions, as well as the development of new integrated healthcare degrees and physician certificate education programs.

Dr. O'Donnell has over 4 years of experience as a consultant, trainer, and lecturer in China and Southeast Asia. He continues long-standing physician training programs in Beijing and has presented many other training sessions in Shanghai, Guangzhou, and Shenzhen. Dr. O'Donnell has presented at conferences in the United States, China, Taiwan, and Malaysia. He has coordinated training visits for Chinese physicians to the United States. He has been a faculty teaching courses at Sichuan University and Beijing Normal University. He is on the editorial board of the journal the *International Journal of Psychotherapy, Counseling & Psychiatry: Theory, Research & Clinical Practice* and also the journal *Family Medicine and Community Health.*

Prior to his current position, Dr. O'Donnell spent over 10 years as a leader in health plans as director of disease management programs. He directed teams of physicians, nurses, dieticians, and behavioral health consultants on providing patient prevention and disease management programs for conditions such as hypertension, diabetes, and depression. He has consulted with national companies on the design, implementation, and evaluation of health management programs that incorporate web-based patient education and self-management tools. He is a leader in the application of phone and table apps for health management outcomes and behavior change for patients with chronic illness.

Earlier in his career he served as director of outpatient behavioral health clinics that were connected with the patient community health clinic and family physician. He provided physician consultation and training on behavioral health problems. Earlier he was director of psychiatric hospital inpatient units. He trained psychiatrists and nurses on behavioral health and launched a comprehensive group education treatment program for patients with severe mental illness. Dr. O'Donnell has significant experience treating the severely mentally ill, including as a community-based care manager providing crisis management. His clinical experience includes treatment of adult depression, anxiety, and trauma, substance abuse, child treatment of attention deficient disorder, autism spectrum disorders and oppositional defiant disorders, and adolescent treatment for family conflict, substance abuse, and school behavior problems. He is experienced in individual, couples and family, and group psychotherapy treatment techniques.

Dr. O'Donnell has dedicated his career to the delivery of healthcare programs that improve patient satisfaction and clinical outcomes while also improving cost-efficiency. He has blended a career that combines deep management and clinical experience. He has a successful track record in academic education with the highly successful Doctor of Behavioral Health program. Finally, he has developed an extensive catalog of education and training programs designed specifically for the China and Southeast Asia healthcare system.

Felicia Trembath is currently with Arizona State University as a postdoctoral researcher and faculty associate with the programs in Integrated Behavioral Health in the College of Health Solutions. She also currently serves on the executive board for the Arizona Public Health Association. She previously served as a fellow with the Health Systems Integration Program (HSIP) through CDC/CSTE and worked on integrating health information across health systems throughout Maricopa County, Arizona.

Dr. Trembath has a PhD in Epidemiology and an MPH from Purdue University. During her graduate work at Purdue University she taught courses and conducted research into public health issues. As a Vista Volunteer with Americorps in Sheridan, Wyoming, she worked with the Coordinated School Health program to develop healthy school teams at local schools and administer the fluoride rinse program to elementary students. Dr. Trembath also worked with the Wyoming Department of Health as a field epidemiologist stationed in Sheridan, Wyoming, where she conducted routine disease investigations statewide and assisted with investigations of outbreaks of Salmonella and Norwalk virus.

Section I
Introduction

Chapter 1
Introduction

Rodger Kessler and C. R. Macchi

Background and Need

This volume focuses on emerging workforce development initiatives designed to support understanding and practice of the following dimensions of integrated care:

- Population health management
- An integrated medical behavioral health budget and payment system
- Tailoring knowledge and training to ACA and Triple Aim implications
- Measuring levels of integration and relationship to outcomes
- Key objectives to guide the development, implementation, and evaluation of training outcomes

Learning Objectives of This Chapter

Trainees will:

1. List and discuss the evolution of primary care-based behavioral health from the Affordable Care Act (ACA) framework.
2. Identify the changes inherent in a carve-in and pay-for-quality model of care.
3. Contrast the elements of population care compared to individual-focused care.
4. Outline a business case for behavioral health integration.
5. Propose a continuous quality improvement (CQI) project focused on some element of integrated primary care.

R. Kessler (✉) · C. R. Macchi
Integrated Behavioral Health Programs, College of Health Solutions,
Arizona State University, Phoenix, AZ, USA
e-mail: rodger.kessler@asu.edu; crmacchi@asu.edu

C. R. Macchi, R. Kessler (eds.), *Training to Deliver Integrated Care*,
https://doi.org/10.1007/978-3-319-78850-0_1

6. List the dimensions of Peek's Lexicon of Collaborative Care, and review how the dimensions are measured by the Practice Integration Profile (PIP).
7. Discuss a rapid, actionable, and valid evaluation method for Primary Care Behavioral Health (PCBH), and use RE-AIM dimensions to apply the evaluation method to the CQI project identified earlier.

Behavioral Care as Part of a Primary Care-Centric Triple Aim-Focused Healthcare

There are at least two contemporary drivers focusing healthcare. The first is the Affordable Care Act (ACA), and its redefinition of healthcare priorities focused around whole-person care, with primary care at the center. In addition, the cornerstones of care include a focus on accomplishing the Triple Aims of healthcare-improved patient experience, improved outcomes, and bending the curve of the overall costs of care. The ACA shifts the focus of healthcare delivery models from care for individual to population-focused care. There is a targeted focus on clinical and cost outcomes. Team-based, whole-person care is directly acknowledged and supported. Training becomes inter-professional to support a team-based workforce.

Training has traditionally focused on what practitioners *do* rather than on the *results* of their efforts. The recent changes shift the focus toward thinking and learning skills concentrated on changing patient outcomes and data-driven healthcare decisions. Systems of care become crucial. In a primary care behavioral model, we can predict that a certain percentage of patients need non-primary care-based behavioral services. Usually linkages have been haphazard or nonexistent. Non-primary care-based behavioral practitioners have a crucial role and also need to be trained in the primary care model to optimize participation in that role.

The second contemporary healthcare reform driver is a population health management (PHM) approach to service delivery. Systems of care are focused on identifying and addressing patient populations with co-occurring medical and behavioral issues. This broad-based approach aims to improve the efficient use of limited resources while increasing the reach and impact of targeted interventions. The identification of patient populations and patient need is predicated on the use of and reporting from data management systems. Often referred to as "big data," these systems collect patient medical data from electronic health records (EHR) and other sources that, when extracted and analyzed, highlight the healthcare needs of broad patient populations. The results transform into clinical pathways, development and delivery of targeted interventions, and improved quality of healthcare delivery and patient outcomes.

Behavioral Health (BH): From Carve-Out to Carve-In

Historically medical care and behavioral care have been separate clinical, organizational, and financial system. Behavioral health has traditionally operated in its own healthcare silo. These issues have not yet been systematically addressed in healthcare reform, though there are many efforts to generate ways to work around the barriers to cobble together some form of primary care integration. This history and current state have consequences.

We have trained behavioral health clinicians to these differences. This has resulted in many collaborative and integrated efforts functioning as carve-outs inside of primary care, with clinicians untrained in the culture, organization, and skills necessary to practice in integrated settings. Training BH practitioners for a carve-in approach to integrated healthcare begins with highlighting the overlapping behavioral knowledge and skills with the other members of the medical team. Rather than simply adding a BH specialist to the medical team, the nature of the team adjusts by carving in behavioral dimensions of patient care. Training must address systems-level change that supports a biopsychosocial (Engel, 1980) approach within each team member's scope of practice. Within this context, BH practitioner training focuses on developing specialized knowledge and skills that complement existing roles while addressing patient's complex behavioral health needs.

Population Health Management (PHM) Initiatives and Programs

Chapter 4 details a shift of focus on individual patients to populations of patients such as all patients in the practice panel with asthma or with asthma and have high ER use. This is a healthcare system shift, not unique to behavioral health. In fact, despite an abundant health psychology and behavioral medicine literature supporting behavioral treatments for a broad variety of patient populations currently, there is little behavioral population health activity, and it has not been the focus of contemporary behavioral and medical collaborative care or integration efforts. Nonetheless, to practice in primary care requires knowledge and skills associated with this change. The treatment of diabetes is as much a focus of panel-based integration as the treatment of depression. Data-driven PHM must be embedded in electronic health records and requires collection of patient reported outcomes. The primary role of behavioral health within primary care focuses on the assessment and intervention of the biopsychosocial aspects of medical presentations and disease.

Business of Healthcare Management

Behavioral care as part of medicine is intuitively a good idea; however, behavioral health is now in the healthcare business. No money, no mission! Integrating and conducting behavioral health in primary care rests first on the business case, second on clinical utility. Generating the business case requires data to make the initial case and more data to demonstrate continued effectiveness. The effective, efficient, efficacious incorporation of the business of healthcare management with the development, implementation, and evaluation of healthcare delivery is part of the BH task.

Training must include addressing the interconnected dimensions (i.e., clinical, operational, and financial) of care (Peek, 2009). Decisions focused on one dimension of practice have implications for the other two dimensions. An example: Patients with behavioral health appointments frequently are seen on different days than primary care appointment. This results in higher level of missed appointments; however, if scheduled on the same day, many insurers will not pay for two different billings on the same day! Clinical, operational, and financial perspectives are often different but interdependent!

Healthcare Delivery Is Informed by Applied, Translational Quality Improvement

The delivery of care is an evolving ongoing process between clinician and patient; clinician, patient, and practice; and practice and system. Changes in the one require changes in the other that affect the organization and care delivery processes. Such change in healthcare is informed by continuous quality improvement (CQI) that presents conceptual and operational struggles for the healthcare system, *not* a technology issue. Learning and implementing continuous quality improvement is a skill and organizational development issue.

CQI is a major operational focus of primary care. Behavioral health (BH) clinicians have generally not been trained in continuous quality improvement (CQI) but need to be. Currently behavioral health has not been a large focus of system- and practice-level quality improvement.

Levels of Integration (The Six Dimensions of the PIP)

Behavior care is delivered within primary care in many ways. We have not been able to describe care models in a clear and consistent manner. We know little about whether levels of integration and the varying dimensions that produce different outcomes. For many years, collaborative care or integration has operated in the absence of an identified theory of practice. There had not been an agreed-upon nosology of integrated primary are, but we now do.

In 2013, Peek presented the Lexicon of Collaborative Care (Peek & National Integration Academy Council, 2013). This lexicon is a set of concepts and definitions, developed by expert consensus, which describes what we mean by behavioral health and primary care integration—a functional definition of what things look like in practice. A consensus lexicon enables effective communication and concerted action among clinicians, care systems, health plans, payers, researchers, policymakers, business modelers, and patients working for effective, widespread implementation on a meaningful scale.

While a unifying theory is important, it is not sufficient. One cannot measure theory unless translated into measurement and then assess levels of practice integration efforts. Measurement provides the opportunity to evaluate the levels of integrated practice against other Triple Aim outcomes. The Practice Integration Profile (PIP) is a 30-item, electronically administered measure of integrated care processes. We operationalized Peek's key clauses into six measurable dimensions: practice workflow, clinical services and providers, workspace arrangement, shared care and integration method, case identification, patient engagement and retention, and a total score. We developed item clusters operationalizing each of these dimensions. Further feedback and pilot testing resulted in adjusted language for comprehension and readability. The same process was used to develop a scoring system, which can be used to generate a score for each individual dimension and a practice total score. The current version of the instrument (PIP v5.0) automatically self-scores and can be completed in 10 min (Kessler, 2015; Kessler et al., 2015). This now allows on-the-ground evaluation of integrated care practice development, care delivery, and outcomes related to a care model.

The New Research and Evaluation Paradigm

Most of the readers of this book will have an interest in research and evaluation but want to know about specific practice-related outcomes. We suggest a recently developed evaluation framework, called the 5 Rs (Peek et al., 2014). Research often fails to find its way into practice or policy in a timely way, if at all. Given the current pressure and pace of healthcare change, many authors have recommended different approaches to make healthcare research more relevant and rapid. The "5 R's" is an emerging standard that synthesizes recommendations for care delivery research that (1) is relevant to stakeholders, (2) is rapid and recursive in application, (3) redefines rigor, (4) reports on resources required, and (5) is replicable. These R's of the research process are mutually reinforcing and can be supported by training that fosters collaborative and reciprocal relationships among researchers, implementers, and other stakeholders. In sum, a standard is emerging for research that is both rigorous and relevant. Consistent and bold application will increase the value, timeliness, and applicability of the research enterprise.

In addition, Glasgow et al. (2006) identify the relevant evaluation dimensions that support this new research paradigm. Known by its acronym, RE-AIM, the model identifies patient and practice REACH of an intervention, patient and practice *Effectiveness*, practice *Adoption*, implementation *Fidelity*, and whether the service intervention, program, or treatment *Maintains* expected changes.

Workforce Training and Development

Training the workforce must match current and expected level of integration and support the development of skills necessary for making that transition. The contents of this chapter thus far present a 30,000-foot overview of core training topics needed to prepare trainees for the new workforce. As the field of integrated healthcare moves increasingly toward improving outcomes, so also must training move from a transactional pedagogy that imparts knowledge toward a transformational pedagogy that focuses on the outcomes of the learner's competent practice. Next, we will provide an overview of the critical features and processes of effective training programs that support learning outcomes.

Key Training Objectives and Outcomes

Comprehensive training programs are designed to engage the learner in multiple levels of experience and development (see Fig. 1.1). Beginning with learner exposure to key concepts, models, and practice examples, the learner becomes familiar with the multiple dimensions and the state of the science of the integrated healthcare field. Skill acquisition occurs when the learner is provided opportunities to analyze, synthesize, and apply those concepts to novel situations and practice experiences. Training programs that support the development of core competencies

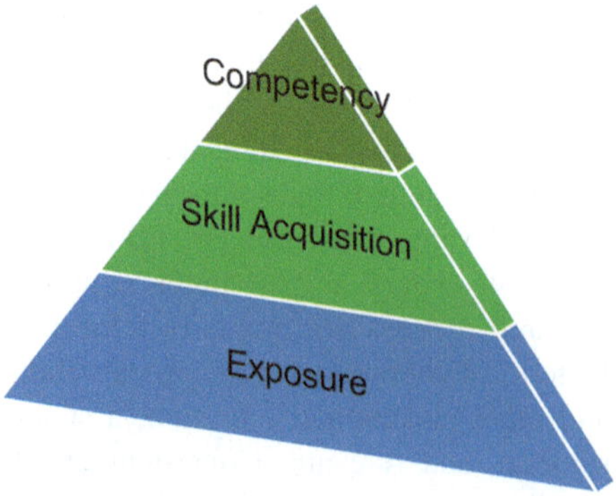

Fig. 1.1 Levels of training objectives

Table 1.1 Example rubric of exposure outcomes

Criterion	Unacceptable	Acceptable	Good	Excellent
Identifies clinical models that are appropriate for the primary care setting	• Lacks identification of a model	• Identifies a model • Does not provide rationale for choice	• Identifies appropriate model • Provides rationale for choice	• Identifies appropriate model • Clearly describes the choice of that model as compared with the range of available models

provide the learner with additional opportunities to repeatedly use and refine skills in the practice environment.

Measuring training outcomes is focused on metrics that provide an expected level of performance for each level of training. Tied to specific behavioral anchors, each metric establishes a standard for that level:

Exposure

Evaluating exposure presents a challenge of determining the level at which the learner understands and applies key concepts and ideas. Training curriculum that exposes a learner is intended to provide that learner with an awareness of the historical development and current state of the science. Measuring the outcomes of this training level requires identifying specific behaviors that reflect the ability to recall, discriminate among terms and concepts, and identify evidences of appropriate use of those ideas. Typically quizzes and exams are used to evaluate the learner's knowledge. Assessment questions are designed to evaluate the learner's ability to define terms, match associated concepts, and identify appropriate applications of those concepts (Table 1.1).

Skill Acquisition

Support of learner skill acquisition moves beyond identification and understanding of content toward the application of knowledge in practice. Learners engaged at this level are expected to analyze, synthesize, and evaluate concepts and then apply those concepts to specific scenarios. Initially, the learner is required to directly apply the concepts and evaluate fit with the scenario. Increasing the level of difficulty occurs when the application of those concepts requires the learner to innovate and adapt to increasingly complex contexts and circumstances (Table 1.2).

Table 1.2 Example rubric of skill development outcomes

Criterion	Unacceptable	Acceptable	Good	Excellent
Identifies clinical models that are appropriate for the primary care setting	• Lacks identification of a model	• Identifies a model • Lacks demonstration of its use	• Demonstrates use of appropriate model • Clearly describes rationale for choice	• Identifies appropriate model • Effectively demonstrates use of the model • Clearly describes the choice of that model for current primary care setting

Table 1.3 Example rubric of competency outcomes

Criterion	Unacceptable	Acceptable	Good	Excellent
Identifies clinical models that are appropriate for the primary care setting	• Unable to identify needed system-level changes • Identifies a model • Lacks demonstration of model use	• Clearly describes needed system-level changes • Demonstrates use of appropriate model	• Clearly describes needed system-level changes • Identifies limitations of chosen model • Effectively demonstrates adaptation of the model	• Clearly describes needed system-level changes • Identifies limitations of chosen model • Effectively demonstrates adaptations of the model for system-level change • Clearly describes the adaptations of the model for current primary care setting • Specifies an evaluation plan for measuring system-level change

Competency

Training that supports the development of core competencies focuses on learner engagement in system-level change and integrated team-based care. Training curriculum focuses on active skill refinement applied within novel practice contexts. Learners at this level are evaluated based upon the consistent demonstration and adaptation of skills used to work collaboratively with teams to assess, implement, and evaluate system-level changes (Table 1.3).

References

Engel, G. (1980). The clinical application of the biopsychosocial model. *American Journal of Psychiatry,* 131–135.

Glasgow, R. E., Nelson, C. C., Strycker, L. A., & King, D. K. (2006). Using RE-AIM metrics to evaluate diabetes self-management support interventions. *American Journal of Preventative Medicine, 30*, 67–73.

Kessler, R. (2015). Evaluating the process of mental health and primary care integration: The Vermont Integration Profile. *Family Medicine and Community Health, 3*(1), 63–65.

Kessler, R., van Eeghan, C., Mullin, D., Auxier, A., Macchi, C. R., & Littenberg, B. (2015). Measuring behavioral health integration in primary care settings. *Health Psychologist.*

Peek, C. J., Glasgow, R. E., Stange, K. C., Klesges, L. M., Purcell, E. P., & Kessler, R. S. (2014). The 5 R's: An emerging bold standard for conducting relevant research in a changing world. *Annals of Family Medicine, 12*(5), 447–455. https://doi.org/10.1370/afm.1688.

Peek, C. J., & National Integration Academy Council. (2013). *Lexicon for behavioral health and primary care integration: Concepts and definitions developed by expert concensus.* Rockville, MD: AHRQ Publication Retrieved from http://integrationacademy.ahrq.gov/sites/default/files/Lexicon.pdf.

Peek, C. J. (2009). Integrating care for persons not only disease. *Journal of Clinical Psychology in Medical Settings, 16*(1), 16–20.

Section II
Overview of Integration: State of the Science

Chapter 2
Integrated Behavioral Healthcare Models

Colleen Clemency Cordes, Jeff Reiter, and Lesley Manson

Key Historical Shifts That Influenced Integrated Care Development

The past 30 years has been marked by a proliferation of practice models and research related to integrated behavioral health in primary care (Archer et al., 2012; Babor et al., 2007; Beehler, Funderburk, Possemato, & Dollar, 2013; Blount, 1998; Collins, Hewson, Munger, & Wade, 2010; Kathol, deGruy, & Rollman, 2014; Katon et al., 1995; Kessler, 2015; Peek, Cohen, & deGruy, 2014; Robinson & Reiter, 2016; Yano, Bair, Carrasquillo, Krein, & Rubenstein, 2014). Multiple shifts have occurred in an effort to pave the way for the paradigm of integrated behavioral healthcare as practiced (in its various forms) today; however, explicit efforts to train the workforce of the future have typically lagged behind emerging policy and practice models (Blount & Miller, 2009; Hall et al., 2015; McDaniel et al., 2014; Serrano, Cordes, Cubic & Daub, 2018; Strosahl, 2005).

As with many large and involved trends, tracing the journey of integrated care back to a specific source is probably not possible; multiple forces have converged over time to propel and shape the journey, each working synergistically with the others. However, one clear early catalyst was research done in the late 1960s (Follette & Cummings, 1967; Cummings & Follette, 1968) that demonstrated for the first time the economic value that even brief behavioral interventions can have. This research, conducted at Kaiser Permanente in California, showed that just one to six psychotherapy visits reduced the medical utilization of patients to such an extent that the costs of providing the therapy were easily offset. The results not only

C. C. Cordes (✉) · J. Reiter · L. Manson
Integrated Behavioral Health Programs, College of Health Solutions,
Arizona State University, Phoenix, AZ, USA
e-mail: Colleen.Clemency@asu.edu; jreiter1@asu.edu; lesley.manson@asu.edu

C. R. Macchi, R. Kessler (eds.), *Training to Deliver Integrated Care*,
https://doi.org/10.1007/978-3-319-78850-0_2

provided the first good evidence of the cost-offset opportunities of behavioral care but also rattled the traditional therapy world by showing that such results could be obtained in just a few visits.

A bit later, George Engel's work on the biopsychosocial model of care (BPS) marked a turning point in our understanding of the critical synergies between biological, psychological, and social/cultural factors that influence the presentation of chronic illness (Engel, 1977). Engel's BPS model, while controversial at the time, closely aligns with much medical training today. Doctors of osteopathic medicine (DOs) are trained that the "body is a unit and the person is a unit of body, mind, and spirit" and healthcare in general is focusing more on psychosocial factors (Fava & Sonino, 2008). Integrated behavioral healthcare explicitly allows for the delivery of patient-centered care using evidence-based treatments of such factors in the primary care environment (Smith, Fortin, Dwamena, & Frankel, 2013).

Emerging research in the 1980s further supported the need to develop collaborative relationships between primary care and mental health professionals. Psychosocial issues were being increasingly recognized as a major driver of healthcare visits, especially in primary care (Wetzler & Cruess, 1985; Kroenke & Mangelsdorff, 1989), and more research from the Cummings group (noted above) showed the medical cost offset that can result from collaboration between medical and mental health providers. Specifically, the Cummings group partnered with the State of Hawaii and the Health Care Financing Administration to conduct a study called the "Hawaii Project." This study randomized almost 130,000 Medicaid and federal employee patients to either healthcare as usual or to an experimental condition in which physical and mental healthcare were tightly coordinated. The results of this prospective, controlled study punctuated the earlier findings of the Cummings group, showing an impressive 20–30% reduction in medical costs for patients in the experimental group, even after accounting for the costs of psychotherapy (Cummings, Dorken, Pallak, & Henke, 1991; Laygo et al., 2003).

The results from the Hawaii Project emerged at around the same time that an awakening of sorts was occurring regarding the nature of mental health treatment in the USA. In response to the 1978 President's Commission on Mental Health, the National Institute of Mental Health initiated in the 1980s large national surveys of the prevalence and incidence of psychiatric problems and of the distribution of care for those problems. To the astonishment of many, the data that emerged from these surveys not only showed psychiatric conditions to be very common (Regier et al., 1984; Kessler et al., 1994) but also showed that the majority of services for these conditions is delivered in primary care (Regier et al., 1993). The surprising data provided perhaps the strongest catalyst for jump-starting the integration movement, highlighting the inadequacy of the specialty mental health sector and dubbing primary care the "de facto mental health care system" of the country (Regier et al., 1993).

Spurred on by these findings, behavioral health providers began locating themselves inside willing primary care clinics, in an attempt to bring their treatment to the place where it was most needed. Many were also already in primary care, as behavioral science faculty in family medicine residency programs, but had previously been more focused on educating future physicians than on practicing themselves in clinics. As the impetus for integration grew, these early pioneers brought what they knew to primary care; they mostly practiced a "colocated therapy" model, providing traditional psychotherapy inside of primary care (see Blount [1998], for a description of this as well as other approaches). Their influence was profoundly important for paving the way for the future evolution of integrated care, but in the 1980s and 1990s, their numbers were relatively small.

Meanwhile, with the spotlight increasingly focused on primary care, concerns began to emerge about the quality of care provided by primary care physicians (PCP) for psychiatric issues. Primary care treatment for depression in particular became a focus of study, given the high prevalence of depression, as well as the higher medical costs, higher care utilization, and significant functional disability associated with the condition. A 1993 review by the Agency for Health Care Policy and Research (AHCPR; now known as the Agency for Healthcare Research and Quality, or AHRQ) acknowledged the importance of primary care-based treatment of depression but also warned of the paucity of data supporting such treatment (Depression Guideline Panel, 1993). At the same time, other research was documenting the frequent under-recognition of depression in primary care, as well as the frequent inappropriate and/or inadequate use of antidepressants (Keller & Lavori, 1988; Katon & Schulberg, 1992).

All of this was occurring just as antidepressant treatment of depression was exploding in volume, especially in primary care. The emergence of SSRI antidepressant medications in the 1980s revolutionized pharmacotherapy for depression because of the safer and lower side effect profile of SSRIs. This allowed primary care physicians to prescribe more comfortably and hence more liberally. Primary care providers now prescribe an overwhelming majority of antidepressants in the country (Mark, Levit, & Buck, 2009; Pratt, Brody, & Gu, 2011).

With all of this as a backdrop, a good deal of research and clinical innovation was launched in the 1980s and 1990s with the goal of improving depression outcomes in primary care through improved antidepressant prescribing practices. The most prolific and influential of this work was done at the University of Washington Medical School, by a team led by the psychiatrist Wayne Katon. In their early work, the Katon team showed that treatment outcomes could be improved by placing psychiatrists in primary care, where they conducted patient education and alternated visits with the PCP to collaboratively manage patients (Katon et al., 1995).

Yet, for all of the challenges of getting effective medication treatment to patients in primary care, the team also realized that even fewer patients were receiving behavioral interventions. Randomized controlled trials (RCTs) of behavioral interventions in primary care had shown some promise, but rarely were such services provided (Brown & Schulberg, 1995). Thus, inspired by their results with psychiatrists focused mostly on improving medication management, the Katon team decided to explore whether outcomes could be similarly improved using non-psychiatrists focused mostly on improving the delivery of behavioral (i.e., non-medication) management of patients.

The seminal study of their effort was a RCT conducted by Katon et al. (1996). This study utilized a psychologist who provided behavioral interventions to patients with depression while also helping oversee the PCP's management of antidepressant medications (with the supervision of a psychiatrist). However, in contrast to the traditional long-term psychotherapy approach that had mostly been used up to that time in both primary care and specialty settings (Brown & Schulberg, 1995), the behavioral component in this study was brief (4–6 visits, most of which lasted 30 min). The briefer approach was tried in response to the high attrition rate of long-term therapy in primary care (Brown & Schulberg, 1995) as well as the promising results of brief therapy in other studies (Mynors-Wallis, Gath, Lloyd-Thomas, & Tomlinson, 1995; Schulberg et al., 1993). Results of this important study showed that, compared to patients receiving usual primary care treatment, the intervention patients achieved better care outcomes and also adhered better to antidepressant medications.

With publication of these early studies, the University of Washington team set the stage for the next step in the evolution of integrated primary care. The research team led by Katon split into two camps, one remaining at the university to focus mostly on refining the medication approach to integration and the other leaving to focus mostly on disseminating the behavioral approach.

The university-based, psychiatry-led group obtained funding for a large RCT of 1801 depressed older adults spread over 18 primary care clinics. Led by psychiatrist Jurgen Unutzer, this trial randomly assigned depressed older adults to either primary care treatment as usual or to a collaborative/stepped-care disease management program run inside primary care. Titled "Improving Mood – Promoting Access to Collaborative Treatment" ("IMPACT"), this study showed that collaborative care doubled the effectiveness of usual depression care, improved patient and provider satisfaction, and was also more cost-effective (Unutzer et al., 2002; Katon et al., 2005). A number of subsequent studies have achieved similar results, typically for patients with depression and anxiety (Katon, Unutzer, Wells, & Jones, 2010).

Today, the approach to integration used in the IMPACT study is typically called the "Collaborative Care Model," or "CoCM." The model, a refinement of the original approach described in Katon et al. (1995), took much of its form from the work of a second research team based out of Seattle. This second team, led by internist Ed Wagner, MD, from Group Health Cooperative (a regional managed care organization), actually included some staff who were also involved in IMPACT. The Wagner team was working on a different approach to organizing primary care for a variety of chronic conditions and eventually developed what became known as the "Chronic Care Model" (Wagner, Austin, & Von Korff, 1996; Wagner et al., 2001). The emphasis of the Chronic Care Model is on developing a team approach that includes an allied health professional such as a nurse who provides close monitoring and frequent contacts with patients.

The influence of the Chronic Care Model on the CoCM is a clear one, as the latter includes many key components of the former (Katon et al., 2010). The CoCM relies on enhanced patient education, a standardized outcome tracking tool, and use of a registry to track various aspects of the patient's care. A central member of the

CoCM team is an allied health professional such as a nurse or behavioral health provider, called a "care manager," who provides close monitoring and follow-up of patients (often via phone). A consulting psychiatrist oversees the care of these care managers and also recommends, as needed, any changes to the antidepressant prescribing of the PCP.

The CoCM is now utilized in many primary care organizations around the country as at least one part of integration efforts. Recently, the Centers for Medicare and Medicaid Services (CMS) developed new codes to help pay organizations for use of the model, which should help ensure its continued use (information regarding the codes can be found here: https://www.cms.gov/Medicare/Medicare-Fee-for-Service-Payment/PhysicianFeeSched/Downloads/Behavioral-Health-Integration-Fact-Sheet.pdf). For more information regarding the model, visit www.aims.uw.edu. The website is run by a center called "Advancing Integrated Mental Health Solutions," or the "AIMS Center," based at the University of Washington. The AIMS Center is run by the psychiatrist who led the IMPACT trial (Jurgen Unutzer) and is the organization most commonly associated with the CoCM; researching, consulting, and disseminating CoCM are its primary function.

As mentioned earlier, development of the CoCM was spurred mostly by members of the Katon-led group who focused first and foremost on improving the delivery of antidepressant medications in primary care. Two other members of that group, psychologists Patricia Robinson and Kirk Strosahl, left to pursue integration from a different angle. Robinson had been the second author on the Katon group's RCT of behaviorally focused primary care interventions (Katon et al., 1996), while Strosahl was at nearby Group Health Cooperative (the same organization that employed the Wagner team, though Strosahl conducted clinical work at Group Health and research with the Katon team). Robinson and Strosahl were largely interested in disseminating behavioral interventions more broadly; so, whereas the Katon group focused mostly on improving medication use in primary care and less on behavioral strategies, Robinson and Strosahl did the reverse.

In addition to having a different focus in their integration efforts, these two groups also used different strategies to advance their respective approaches to integration. The Katon group remained at the university, continuing to research the collaborative care approach, gathering data to gradually demonstrate for policymakers and healthcare leaders the value of collaborative care. Robinson and Strosahl, in contrast, set out to engage with organizations at the practice level. Spring boarding from the Katon et al. (1996) RTC, they worked with organizations to help them implement the behavioral approach used in that study, which they referred to as a "behavioral consultation" approach (Strosahl, 1996; 1997; 1998). Both groups built momentum for their work over time, albeit through these different processes.

As Robinson and Strosahl worked to disseminate the behavioral consultation approach, separate but parallel processes were underway that ultimately helped refine the approach to its present-day form, called the "Primary Care Behavioral Health" or "PCBH" model. First, in 1996, the Institute of Medicine (IOM) gave a clear definition of primary care, describing it as "the provision of integrated, accessible health care services by clinicians who are accountable for addressing a large majority of personal health needs, developing a sustained partnership with patients, and practicing in the context of family and community" (Institute of Medicine, 1996). In that same publication, the IOM also discussed the "Patient-Centered Medical Home" ("PCMH") as a tool for achieving quality primary care. The PCMH had first been mentioned in 1967 by the American Academy of Pediatrics, but the IOM publication increased its visibility and relevance to all of primary care. The further establishment of the Patient-Centered Medical Home (PCMH) Joint Principles by the American Academy of Family Physicians, American Academy of Pediatrics, American College of Physicians, and American Osteopathic Association in 2007 marked a critical point in the efforts to integrate behavioral health in primary care (American Academy of Family Physicians [AAFP], American Academy of Pediatrics [AAP], American College of Physicians [ACP], and American Osteopathic Association [AOA], 2007). The principles of the PCMH explicitly highlighted the importance of coordinated and/or integrated care across a complex healthcare system (inclusive of behavioral health services) and the patient's community (Baird et al., 2014).

The IOM definition denotes several core features and functions that clearly differentiate primary care from the specialties. It notes that primary care must act as the overseer of every person's health and the gatekeeper to the healthcare system, must understand the context of patients' lives, and must aim for a long-term partnership with patients. In order to meet these lofty goals, primary care providers (PCPs) must practice differently than many specialists. To accommodate so many patients, PCPs must learn to practice quickly and see a high patient volume; they must ask about all aspects of patients' lives and know how to intervene with virtually any problem in patients of any age; and they must understand how to help patients access services and care outside of their own clinic when necessary.

As the behavioral consultation model took hold in primary care clinics around the country, the need for adapting its practices to better fit primary care became clear. Behavioral health providers new to primary care gradually began to understand primary care better and began to grasp the need for behavioral health services that are more accessible and broad than those in the original behavioral consultation model. Whereas the initial model in the 1996 RCT was focused mostly on a relatively small number of depressed patients, the IOM definition made clear that primary care's role is to manage any sort of health condition and to serve the entire population. Thus, the behavioral consultation model began to adapt to these broader needs of primary care. Behavioral health providers practicing in this model began looking for ways to see more patients, with a broader range of problems, in a more accessible fashion.

The innovation of the PCMH lent a hand to this adaptation effort. With its emphasis on team-based care, the PCMH moved primary care away from physician-centric care. Team development became the focus of primary care. This meant that PCPs must learn to distribute their work across a team, but it also meant that other team members must understand the role of primary care and how to contribute to it.

Thus, as the behavioral consultation model spread, the demands of primary care and the PCMH pushed changes in how the model was applied. Early descriptions of the model (Strosahl, 1996, 1997, 1998) focused mostly around the importance of having the BH provider located in the PC clinic, providing briefer interventions than traditional therapy (both in terms of visit length and treatment duration), working closely with the PCP to help improve PCP skill and comfort level with behavioral interventions for depression, and charting in the same medical record. Owing to the nature of the BH provider's involvement and the goal of improving PCP comfort and skill, the BH provider was conceptualized as a "consultant" rather than a "therapist."

To better meet the new demands and team-based orientation of primary care, this early version of the model expanded in a few significant ways. First, the focus on depression was broadened; the same general model was used as a delivery platform for behavioral interventions for a wide range of conditions. Second, an emphasis was placed on access; to meet the needs of the primary care team, the BH provider practiced flexible access, where the goal became always to offer same-day access to patients. Third, high patient volume became a goal. Thus, while the basics of the original model were maintained, the new application made the care broader and more accessible. The new platform provided a way for empirically supported behavioral interventions to be provided for more problems, to more patients, in a more accessible manner.

Today this evolved approach is commonly referred to as the "Primary Care Behavioral Health" (PCBH) model. The first detailed and extensive descriptions of the model came in the mid-2000s (Gatchel & Oordt, 2003; Robinson & Reiter, 2007; Hunter et al., 2009), with further refinements and adaptations published a decade later (Freeman, 2011; Hunter, Goodie, Oordt, & Dobmeyer, 2017; Robinson & Reiter, 2015; Serrano, 2015). As described in a recent publication (Reiter, Dobmeyer, & Hunter, 2017), the model is a team-based approach that aims to make primary care better for the whole population (i.e., both for patients with and without behavioral conditions). The full definition from that publication states that the model is a:

> team-based primary care approach to managing behavioral health problems and biopsychosocially-influenced health conditions. The model's main goal is to enhance the primary care team's ability to manage and treat such problems/conditions, with resulting improvements in primary care services for the entire clinic population. The model incorporates into the primary care team a behavioral health provider, typically referred to as a behavioral health consultant (BHC), to extend and support the primary care provider (PCP) and team. The BHC works as a generalist who provides high volume services that are accessible, team-based, and a routine part of primary care. Specifically, the BHC assists in the care of patients of any age and with any health condition (generalist); engages with a large percentage of the clinic population (high volume); strives to intervene with all patients on the day they are referred (accessible); shares clinic space and resources and assists the team in various ways (team-based); and is a routine part of biopsychosocial care (routine). To accomplish these goals, BHCs use focused (15–30 minute) visits to assist with specific symptoms or functional improvement. Follow-up is based in a consultant approach in which patients are followed by the BHC and PCP until functioning or symptoms begin improving; at that point, the PCP resumes sole oversight of care but re-engages the BHC at any time, as needed. Patients not improving are referred to a higher intensity of care, though if that is not possible the BHC may continue to assist until improvements are noted. This consultant approach also aims to improve the PCP's biopsychosocial management of health conditions in general.

Like the CoCM, the PCBH model is used by many organizations around the country as at least one part of an integration effort. The CoCM and PCBH models actually are often used together, because they are quite complementary (Unutzer, 2016). For example, a strength of the PCBH model is its reach, with the behavioral health provider engaging with a high patient volume and a broad array of problems; but a limitation is that it does not involve the behavioral health provider in treating the patient all the way to target (which means patients can be easily lost to follow-up). Conversely, a strength of the CoCM is that it tracks patients in a registry until treated to target, which minimizes the number lost to follow-up; but a limitation is that it is designed only for treatment of certain conditions, which limits the reach of the model. Thus, having both services available allows for a comprehensive service that meets many needs (Reiter et al., 2018).

Just as the two models have taken different clinical approaches to integration, they also have taken different approaches to dissemination of the model and have faced different challenges. The CoCM was built primarily by university-based researchers who then worked on spreading the model into the clinical world through policy and administrative efforts. However, despite dozens of clinical trials documenting the model's effectiveness, there have often been challenges with implementing it in the real clinical world. Even clinics that participated in the successful research trials often have not maintained the service after completing the trials (Solberg et al., 2013). To further complicate the picture, a large implementation trial of the CoCM in 75 clinics, called the DIAMOND study, found no difference in the depression treatment outcomes of patients enrolled in CoCM compared to those receiving usual care (Crain et al., 2013; Institute for Clinical Systems Improvement, 2014). There have been more positive findings from that trial as well, but the negative findings were from the most rigorous analysis funded by the National Institute of Mental Health (NIMH).

The PCBH model, by contrast, was built primarily by clinicians who spread it at the practice level. Popular with clinicians and patients, the PCBH model grew rather organically to become a widely used approach. For example, it is implemented in every primary care clinic throughout the Department of Defense (Hunter et al., 2014). However, it has been criticized for lacking a research base that clearly demonstrates its value. As of this writing, 29 peer-reviewed studies have examined the PCBH model, but while these have generally produced supportive results, many of the studies have significant methodological concerns that need to be addressed in future research (Hunter et al., 2017). A good source of information about the PCBH model's research and implementation is the website of the PCBH Special Interest Group of the Collaborative Family Healthcare Association (CFHA): http://www.cfha.net/?page=PCBHResources.

While the CoCM and PCBH models may be the most recognizable approaches to integration, few systems seem to use approaches that clearly adhere to one model or another. The field of integrated primary care is really only now beginning to grow significantly and as such is still in search of the model that will best meet the needs of primary care and its patients. To that end, Kathol et al. (2014) have proposed components they believe will result in sustainable and value-added integration.

They argue for an approach that would incorporate on-site or virtual behavioral health teams into primary care, utilizing them in a targeted fashion designed to obtain the most value.

The approach outlined by Kathol et al. (2014) includes seven components. First, they recommend eliminating payer carve-outs for behavioral health services and, instead, combining behavioral and medical benefits into one plan for general medical/surgical benefits. Second, rather than the universal screening commonly done today (e.g., for depression or substance misuse), they recommend screening for such problems only in patients with high-cost and/or high-disability conditions such as diabetes, asthma, and others. Third, they recommend staffing clinics with on-site or virtual behavioral health teams consisting of providers with various degrees and training. Fourth, they suggest using those providers in a stepped-care fashion such that patients not improving may be escalated to care that is more intensive and/or provided by someone with a higher level of training. The goal with this step is to use limited behavioral health resources in the most efficient fashion. The fifth component focuses on treating conditions that are known to be high cost but reversible (e.g., depression, diabetes and others) by applying a "treat-to-target" model in which patients are tracked in a registry by a care manager who helps ensure they are followed until symptoms are under control. The regular use of standardized treatment outcome tools to help gauge the success (or lack thereof) of treatment is also key to this approach. Sixth, they emphasize the application of higher-intensity behavioral interventions over the more commonly encountered counseling interventions, for patients with significant behavioral health needs. Seventh, they advocate for the use of care coordinators who can help patients navigate the various medical and social service systems to obtain the help they need. Kathol et al. (2014) recognize that there are a number of barriers to systems initiating an approach such as this at the current time, but their intent is more to lay a foundation for what they believe should be the next step in the evolution of integrated care. As with each of the approaches discussed here, time will tell where the data and the policies take us; about the only guarantee is that integration will in fact continue to change over time as the field learns and grows.

IBH Training Initiatives

As models of integrated care emerged, so did efforts to develop this burgeoning workforce; these efforts are described in detail in Chaps. 9 and 11. The history of integrated behavioral health training began to accelerate in the late 1990s in concert with the expanded recognition of behavioral care needs in primary care (see Appendix), and training has evolved to meet the growing demands of the emerging workforce. Initial efforts to train behavioral health providers in team-based care approaches were focused on the development of texts that could be adopted as "training manuals" for on-the-job training, such as Robinson and Reiter's (2015) *Behavioral Consultation in Primary Care*, which articulated the role of a behavioral health consultant as part of the primary care team. Additional publications recognized that many behavioral health providers from diverse backgrounds (i.e., marriage and family therapy, counseling, social work, and psychology) lacked an understanding of the role of behavior in chronic disease and focused on the provision of knowledge and skills pertaining to chronic disease management (Hunter et al., 2009, 2017; deGruy, Dickinson, & Staton, 2002; James & O'Donohue, 2009). These publications provided guidance on the development of adaptive strategies and techniques to address health behavior change and motivational enhancement to effectively address health conditions commonly treated in primary care. More recently, texts have begun to emerge to address the administrative aspects of integrated behavioral health (e.g., financing, workflows, documentation) that are critical to the long-term success of behavioral health programs (Corso, Hunter, Dahl, Kallenberg, & Manson, 2016).

Despite these texts, it was clear that existing training efforts were insufficient to support the needs of the workforce. In 2007, the University of Massachusetts launched the first web-based training program for interprofessional teams on the provision of integrated primary care behavioral health (Blount & Miller, 2009). This training program consisted of 36 h of didactic and interactive training that focused primarily on (1) orienting the behavioral health provider to the culture of primary care, (2) adapting the behavioral health provider role in diverse primary care settings, (3) adapting evidence-based approaches to the primary care environment, and (4) incorporating care management as part of a comprehensive approach to patient care. The success of this program, which continues to train a significant number of behavioral health providers and integrated care team members, coincided with increased acceptance of, and evidence in support of, online learning as a viable training modality (U.S. Department of Education, 2010), and the program itself has evolved to include on-demand educational modules with opportunities for live interaction with program faculty during question and answer sessions (http://www.umassmed.edu/cipc/pcbh/overview/).

Subsequent discipline-specific efforts responded to the emerging workforce need by enhancing training programs. For example, the American Psychological Association established a training task force, which published its recommendations for the first time in 2011 (Cubic et al., 2011). This task force highlighted the significant challenge associated with training behavioral health providers in the absence of a consistent model of integration achieving universal acceptance and a rapidly evolving field.

The Doctor of Behavioral Health (DBH) program in the College of Health Solutions at Arizona State University opened its doors in 2009, with the goal of training the non-guild-specific integrated behavioral health workforce of the future (chs.asu.edu/dbh). The first of its kind, this program initially set forth to train providers in the domains of medical literacy, evidence-based practice, and healthcare systems and financing, in order to better meet the needs of the evolving integrated care environment. In recent years, the DBH program at ASU launched a management concentration of its degree, focused on additionally training healthcare administrators to oversee practice transformation efforts to further implement integrated care. At the time of this writing, there are approximately 250 graduates from ASU's DBH program, and two other DBH programs have emerged in the USA; two graduate certificates will additionally be launched in Spring 2018 in an effort to further develop the IBH workforce.

While training has evolved, it has often done so without clearly establishing training objectives for work in integrated primary care, and there is not a single set of widely accepted core competencies for behavioral health practice. Over the past 5 years, there have been a number of published competencies for integrated primary care, including those established by the American Psychological Association (APA, 2015), the Substance Abuse and Mental Services Association and the Health Resources and Services Administration (SAMHSA-HRSA) Center for Integrated Health Solutions (Hoge, Morris, Laraia, Pomerantz, & Farley, 2014), and the Eugene S. Farley, Jr. Health Policy Center (Miller et al., 2016), among others. While these competencies share core values of team-based care, collaboration, and evidence-based practice, there is lack of consensus on the critical training domains for, and performance metrics to assess, work in primary care.

How to Select a Model of Integration: Key Concepts for Consideration

It is clear that the selection and implementation of an integration model are multi-faceted processes and require a conceptual frame beyond "let's just go out and hire someone." If there is agreement that the purpose of integration is to improve the quality of care delivered, then a starting point is Donabedian's dimensions of quality of care reflected in his structure-process-outcomes model (2011). To achieve quality of care, integration models must provide structural elements to operate within, a set of processes to operationalize care delivery, and a population of patients and targeted outcomes for those patients to then measure.

The knowledge of the historical development of integrated models and their clinical approaches may be useful in considering the selection of a model of integration, but more important is the evolution of a model that best fits an integrated healthcare program or system. As described earlier, a meta-analysis of studies on integrated care found the strongest outcomes with CoCM and team-based approaches in which primary care providers, care managers, and mental/behavioral health providers coordinate care (Asarnow, Rozenman, Wiblin, & Zeltzer, 2015, Gerrity, 2016; Collins et al., 2010). It may appear to be a simple decision to integrate care; however, there are a number of essential key elements and steps to consider when evaluating an integrated care model for implementation.

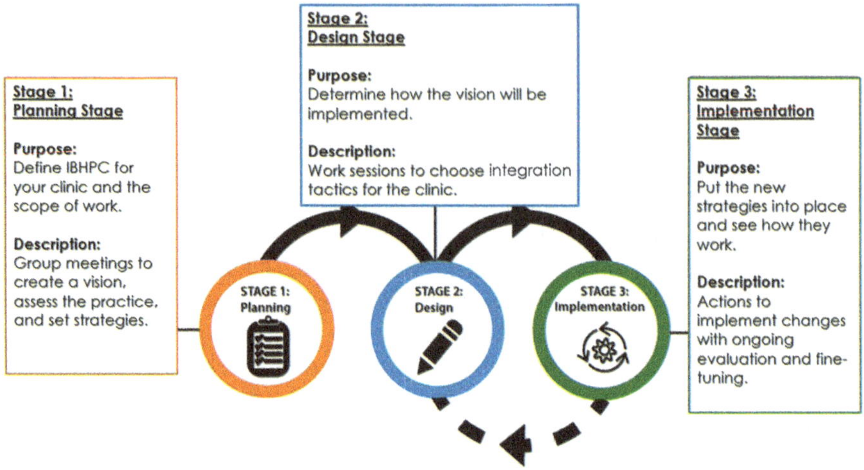

Fig. 2.1 Stages of integrating a model of care. (van Eeghen et al., 2017)

It is important to understand and prioritize the stages of developing a local or system integration model. There are three stages: phase one (planning stage), phase two (design stage), and stage three (implementation and evaluation stage) (see Fig. 2.1). In the planning stage, healthcare systems identify a design team consisting of executives, clinical providers, patients, and staff members who assess need, set parameters of the intervention, and identify resources and actions that will set the structure to develop a model of care. During the design phase, a facilitated team creates the practice's vision of integration; assesses facilitators and barriers, readiness for change, and integration (such as identifying current integrated care functioning and identification of opportunities and challenges related to integrated care); and develops an implementation strategy and plan, complete with tasks, people to execute them, and time frames.

In the final steps of the design stage, the team determines how the vision will be implemented with knowledge of the specific strategies for integrated care and the chosen model. Work sessions focus on tactics for implementation, infrastructure changes needed, and integrated care culture development. Once stage two is complete, the task moves to stage three: implementation and monitoring. This stage translates the design teams' efforts into practice, implementing the plan, creating practice workflows, and using an ongoing data-focused monitoring method to evaluate utility, effectiveness, and efficiency of the intervention. It is important to emphasize that the effort does not have a finish point, rather there need to be ongoing quality improvement and assurance activities as systematic processes to continue to refine structure, process, and outcomes of care.

Tools such as the Practice Integration Profile (PIP; Macchi, Kessler, Auxier, Juvena, & Mullin, 2016) may assist the implementation team to identify current integration functioning. The data from each PIP domain enables the team to select strategies for integration planning and implementation, identification of patient population focus areas (e.g., diabetes, hypertension, depression, insomnia, persistent pain), scope of practice (e.g., capabilities, roles, and responsibilities), service selection (e.g., brief evidence-based interventions, screening, and care coordination), provider participation (e.g., identify the team), culture changes, practice requirements (e.g., shared space/office, electronic health records, infrastructure, billing, and training), and communication planning (e.g., shared communication and documentation). The resulting plan prepares the design team to work together to complete stages toward implementation. These strategies provide guidance for aligning specific training strategies with specific models of integrated care (see Table 2.1).

Conclusion

Multiple practice model shifts have occurred over the past three decades leading us to the integrated behavioral healthcare paradigm. It is critical that policy and practice align to reduce barriers and enhance opportunities for such team-based, collaborative care. Healthcare educational programming, curricula, and workforce training (i.e., skill development, retraining) must be aligned with these burgeoning models of care. For sustainability, training should focus on population health management and the Quadruple Aim of healthcare (Bodenheimer & Sinsky, 2014) with the support of value-based programming and payment models.

Healthcare systems should consider the available resources when choosing and implementing a model, as well as selecting appropriate training opportunities. Training directors should consider whether the clinic has access to skilled BHPs within their organization or need to recruit outside providers to build their interprofessional team. Once an organization identifies and decides to adopt a specific model of integrated care, training needs can be identified through reviewing the distinguishing characteristics and strategies (see Table 2.1). Further, it is beneficial to design training reflective of team-based skills required in primary care (see Chap. 3), population health management skills (see Chap. 4), performance on a medical team (see Chap. 6), and integrated ethical, legal, and professional considerations (Chap. 12).

Table 2.1 Strategies linked to models of integrated care

Strategy for integration	Referral-based and colocated care	Collaborative care (CoCM)	Primary care behavioral health (PCBH)
Problem scope	Narrow	Narrow	Wide
Continuum focus	Acute, chronic	Chronic	Prevention, acute, and chronic
Age scope	Narrow	Narrow	Wide
Ownership of care	Therapist	PCP	PCP
PCP involvement	Low	Low	High
Access to care	Low	Variable	High
Care termination	To target	To target	Improving
Care tracking	No	Yes	Mostly no
Accessibility	Scheduled	On-demand and scheduled	On-demand and scheduled
Dimension	Colocated mental health services	Collaborative care	Team based, flexible
Model of care	Patient based	Population based	Population based
Service delivery structure	Specialized referral	Specialized and consult driven	Primary care driven
Team structure	Specialist	Specialist (on- and off-site)	Part of primary care team
Collaboration	Minimal collaboration Basic collaboration at distance or on-site	Basic collaboration Close collaboration on-site with some system integration	Full collaboration in merged practice with system integration
Primary goals	Management of mental health conditions	Management of mental health conditions Management of comorbid mental and medical health conditions	Promote medical provider/team efficacy and efficiency Support small patient change efforts longitudinally Same-day access Generalist (any age or problem) High patient volume

(continued)

Table 2.1 (continued)

Strategy for integration	Referral-based and colocated care	Collaborative care (CoCM)	Primary care behavioral health (PCBH)
Interventions and visit types	Long-term evidence-based and best practice treatments 50-min and above interventions and visits Specialized assessment Full psychosocial intake Individual, family, and group interventions	Long-term evidence-based treatments; treated to target 30–60-min visits Specialized assessment Full psychosocial intake Individual, population, and group interventions Registry-based tracking Psychiatric oversight and consulting (off-site)	Brief evidence-informed/based treatments and interventions 15–30-min visits and interventions Consultative Educational efforts for the team Individual, population, family, and group interventions Population health management Care pathways
Physical space	Colocated or close proximity (building nearby)	Colocated or close proximity Telehealth	In primary care team Office sharing with medical team
Confidentiality, consent, and documentation	Separate documentation Separate electronic health record (EHR) Shared records with release and consent	Separate documentation Shared or separate EHR	Unified medical record documentation Shared electronic health record Consent is standardized as part of primary care services
Billing and finances	Behavioral health provider billing	Cost-saving focus Behavioral health provider billing Some CCM codes billed by medical provider	Return on investment focus Cost-saving focus Behavioral health provider billing and/or covered as part of primary care services
Provider traits	Specialty knowledge	Specialty knowledge Works well in teams Open to challenge Willing to learn medical terminology	Flexibility Works well in teams Open to challenge Comfortable in fast-paced environments Willing to expand roles and responsibilities for team-based care Willing to learn behavioral medicine and medical terminology

Appendix: IBH Historical Development

Evolution of IBH	Seminal points in the history of IBH publications and training
1600s – Cartesian dualism, which views the mind and body as separate entities, is the prevailing view of health[a]	
1950s – Kaiser Permanente implements the first attempt at integrated (collaborative care) with prepaid psychology contacts	1892 – Andrew Taylor Still founded the American School of Osteopathy, establishing the Doctor of Osteopathic medicine (D.O.) credential. Unlike the previously established M.D., D.O.s are trained to treat the cause of problems, rather than the ramifications of diseases, resulting in a more whole person
1967 – The American Academy of Pediatrics coins the term "medical home" for children with complex needs[b]	
1971 – The term "medical model" is coined by R. D. Laing, who describes it as the "set of procedures in which all doctors are trained"	1969 – Family medicine is recognized as the 20th primary medical subspecialty, resulting in establishment of residency and board certification requirements. Understanding of behavioral science is viewed as a key element of training[j]
1977 – In response to Laing's medical model, Engel publishes in paper on the biopsychosocial model of care, which emphasizes the influence of biological, social, and psychological factors associated with health[c]	
1980s – The "Hawaii Project" demonstrates medical cost offset as a result of collaboration between physicians and mental health providers[d]	
1993 – The Collaborative Family Health Care Coalition (now CFHA) comprised of 15 colleagues from family medicine and family therapy meets for the first time to promote the integration of behavioral health and primary care	1989 – Kroenke and Mangelsdorff publish their article in the *American Journal of Medicine* indicating that the majority of primary care visits are related to behavioral factors (not diagnosed mental health disorders[k])
1996 – IOM defines primary care as the "provision of integrated, accessible healthcare services by clinicians who are accountable for addressing a large majority of personal health needs, developing a sustained partnership with patients, and practicing in the context of family and community[e]"	1991 – The term "evidence-based medicine" emerges and becomes a central focus of medical education 1995 – CFHA holds its first national conference 1995 – Katon publishes his first article on the collaborative care model[l]
1998 – Chronic Care Model (CCM) shifted attention to proactive, population-based approaches to patient chronic care management	
Late 1990s – Several studies are published noting significant differences in the lifespans of patients with severe mental illness	1998 – Alexander Blount publishes his book *Integrated Primary Care: The Future of Medical and Mental Health Collaboration*[m]

(continued)

(continued)

Evolution of IBH	Seminal points in the history of IBH publications and training
2001 – The Institute of Medicine endorses the principle of evidence-based practice	2004 – Frank, McDaniel, Bray, and Heldring publish their edited volume, *Primary Care Psychology*[n]
2006 – The Institute of Medicine articulates the critical need to integrated mental health and substance use in order to achieve quality healthcare[f]	2007 – Patricia Robinson and Jeffrey Reiter publish *Behavioral Consultation and Primary Care: A Guide to Integrating Services*[o]
2007 – The Patient-Centered Medical Home (PCMH) Joint Principles are established[g]	2007 – The University of Massachusetts Medical School launches a distance-learning training program in integrated primary care co-led by behavioral health clinicians and primary care providers[p]
	2008 – Berwick, Nolan, and Whittington describe the Triple Aim[q]
2009 – The World Health Organization launches its Mental Health Gap Action Program (mhGAP), aimed at improving access to evidence-based care in low-income countries by ensuring integration in primary care	2009 – The Interprofessional Education Collaborative (IPEC) is established; it publishes its first set of interprofessional competencies in 2011[r]
	2009 – Hunter and colleagues publish *Integrated Behavioral Health in Primary Care: Step-by-Step Guidance for Assessment and Intervention*[s]
	2009 – The Doctor of Behavioral Health (DBH) program at Arizona State University opens the first doctoral training program exclusively focused on training behavioral health providers in integrated primary care
2010 – The Affordable Care Act is passed, with provisions focused on reimbursement based on quality standards which promote integrated care	2010 – Milbank Memorial Fund publishes its report on *Evolving Models of Behavioral Health Integration in Primary Care*[t]
2010 – The US Department of Veterans Affairs launches its national implementation of Patient Aligned Care Teams (PACT), based on the PCMH[h]	2011- APA Report of the Primary Care Training Task Force is published[u]
	2013 – AHRQ publishes the *Lexicon for Behavioral Health and Primary Care Integration*, providing a shared language for integrated primary care[v]
2014 – The NCQA updates the PCMH Joint Principles to expand the importance and role of integration of behavioral health into the PCMH[i]	2013–present – There is a proliferation of both guild-specific and interprofessional competencies regarding the practice of integrated behavioral health in primary care
	2016 – Corso et al. publish one of the first books focused on challenges with implementing primary care behavioral health[w]
	2017 – NCQA releases 2017 PCMH standards that more specifically articulate the value of behavioral health integration in primary care through the addition of a Behavioral Health Distinction Module[x]

References

[a]Descartes, R., & Moriarty, M. (2008). *Meditations on first philosophy: With selections from the objections and replies*. Oxford, England: Oxford University Press.

[b]Sia, C., Tonniges, T. F., Osterhus, E., & Taba, S. (2004). History of the medical home concept. *Pediatrics, 113*, 1473–1478.

[c]Engle, G. L. (1977). The need for a new medical model: A challenge for biomedicine. *Science, 196*(4286), 129–136.

[d]Cummings, N. S., Dorken, H., Pallak, M. S., & Henke, C. J. (1993). The impact of psychological intervention on health care costs and utilization: The Hawaii Medicaid Project. In N. A. Cummings, & M. S. Pallak (Eds.)., *Medicaid, managed behavioral health and implications for public policy. Volume 2: Healthcare and Utilization Cost Series* (pp. 3–23). San Francisco, CA: Foundation for Behavioral Health.

[e]Institute of Medicine Committee on the future of Primary Care. (1996). *Primary care: America's health in a new era*. Washington, DC: The National Academies Press.

[f]Institute of Medicine. (2006). *Improving the quality of health care for mental and substance-use conditions: Quality chasm series*. Washington, DC: The National Academies Press.

[g]American Academy of Family Physicians, American Academy of Pediatrics, American College of Physicians, & American Osteopathic Association (2007). Joint Principles of the Patient-Centered Medical Home. Retrieved from: http://www.aafp.org/dam/AAFP/documents/practice_management/pcmh/initiatives/PCMHJoint.pdf

[h]Yano, E. M., Bair, M. J., Carrasquillo, O., Krein, S. L., & Rubenstein, L. V. (2014). Patient Aligned Care Teams (PACT): VA's journey to implementing patient-centered medical homes. *Journal of General Internal Medicine, 29*, 547–549.

[i]Baird, M., Blount, A, Brungardt, S., Dickinson, P., Dietrich, A., Epperly, T., et al. (2014). Joint principles: Integrating behavioral health care into the patient-centered medical home. *Annals of Family Medicine, 12*, 183–185.

[j]American Board of Family Medicine. (n.d.). *History of the specialty*. Retrieved from: https://www.theabfm.org/about/history.aspx

[k]Kroenke, K., & Mangelsdorff, A. D. (1989). Common symptoms in ambulatory care: Incidence, evaluation, therapy and outcomes. *American Journal of Medicine, 86*, 262–266. New York, NY: W. W. Norton & Company, Inc.

[l]Katon, W., Von Korff, M., Lin, E., Walker, E., Simon, G. E., Bush, T. et al. (1995). Collaborative management to achieve treatment guidelines. Impact on depression in primary care. *JAMA, 273*, 1026–1031.

[m]Blount, A., (Ed.) (1998). Integrated primary care: The future of medical and mental health collaboration.

[n]Frank, R. G., McDaniel, S. H., Bray, J. H., & Heldring, M. (Eds.) (2004). *Primary care psychology*. Washington, DC: American Psychological Association.

[o]Robinson, P. J., & Reiter, J. T. (2007). *Behavioral consultation and primary care: A guide to integrating services*. New York, NY: Springer.

[p]Blount, A., & Miller, B. F. (2009). Addressing the workforce crisis in integrated primary care. *Journal of Clinical Psychology in Medical Settings, 16*, 113–119.

[q]Berwick, D. M., Nolan, T. W., & Whittington, J. (2008). The Triple Aim: Care, health, and cost. *Health Affairs, 27*(3), 759–769.

[r]Interprofessional Education Collaborative. (n. d.). About the Interprofessional Education Collaborative (IPEC). Retrieved from: https://ipecollaborative.org/About_IPEC.html

[s]Hunter, C. L., Goodie, J. L., Oordt, M. S., & Dobmeyer, A. C. (2009). *Integrated behavioral health in primary care: Step-by-step guidance for assessment and intervention*. Washington, DC: American Psychological Association.

[t]Collins, C., Hewson, D. L., Munger, R., & Wade, T. (2010). *Evolving models of behavioral health integration in primary care*. New York, NY: Milbank Memorial Fund.

[u]Cubic, B., Neumann, C., Kearney, L., McGrath, R., Ruddy, B., Zamudio, A. (2011). Report of the primary care training task force to the APA Board of Educational Affairs. Retrieved from: https://www.apa.org/ed/graduate/task-force-report.pdf

[v]Peek, C. J. and the National Integration Academy Council. (2013). *Lexicon for behavioral health and primary care integration: Concepts and definitions developed by expert consensus*. Rockville, MD: Agency for Healthcare Research and Quality.
[w]Corso, K. A., Hunter, C. L., Dahl, O., Kallenbreg, G. A., & Manson, L. (2016). *Integrating behavioral health into the medical home: A rapid implementation guide*. Phoenix, MD: Greenbranch Publishing.
[x]NCQA. (2017). Patient-centered medical home (PCMH) recognition. Retrieved from: http://www.ncqa.org/programs/recognition/practices/patient-centered-medical-home-pcmh

References

Agency for Healthcare Research and Quality (2011). *Types of quality measures*. Rockville, MD. http://www.ahrq.gov/professionals/quality-patient-safety/talkingquality/create/types.html

American Academy of Family Physicians (AAFP), American Academy of Pediatrics (AAP), American College of Physicians (ACP), & American Osteopathic Association (AOA). (2007). *Joint principles of the patient-centered medical home.* Retrieved from http://www.aafp.org/dam/AAFP/documents/practice_management/pcmh/initiatives/PCMHJoint.pdf

American Psychological Association (2015). *Competencies for psychology practice in primary care.* Retrieved from: http://www.apa.org/ed/resources/competencies-practice.pdf

Archer, J., Bower, P., Gilbody, S., Lovell, K., Richards, D., Gask, L., et al. (2012). Collaborative care for people with depression and anxiety problems. *Cochrane Database of Systematic Reviews,* (10), Art. No.: CD006525. doi: https://doi.org/10.1002/14651858.CD006525.pub2.

Asarnow, J. R., Rozenman, M., Wiblin, J., & Zeltzer, L. (2015). Integrated medical-behavioral care compared with usual primary care for child and adolescent behavioral health: A meta-analysis. *JAMA Pediatrics, 169*(10), 929–937.

Babor, T. F., McRee, B. G., Kassebaum, P. A., Grimaldi, P. L., Ahmed, K., & Bray, J. (2007). Screening, Brief Intervention and Referral to Treatment (SBIRT): Toward a public health approach to the management of substance abuse. *Substance Abuse, 28*(3), 7–30.

Baird, M., Blount, A., Brungardt, S., Dickinson, P., Dietrich, A., Epperly, T., et al. (2014). Development of joint principles: Integrating behavioral health care into the patient-centered medical home. *Annals of Family Medicine, 12*, 183–185.

Beehler, G. P., Funderburk, J. S., Possemato, K., & Dollar, K. M. (2013). Psychometric assessment of the primary care behavioral health provider adherence questionnaire (PPAQ). *Translational Behavioral Medicine, 3*, 379–391.

Blount, A. (1998). *Integrated primary care: The future of medical and mental health collaboration.* New York: Norton Professional Books.

Blount, F. A., & Miller, B. F. (2009). Addressing the workforce crisis in integrated primary care. *Journal of Clinical Psychology in Medical Settings, 16*, 113–119.

Bodenheimer, T., & Sinsky, C. (2014) From Triple to Quadruple Aim: Care of the Patient Requires Care of the Provider. *The Annals of Family Medicine 12*(6), 573–576.

Brown, C., & Schulberg, H. C. (1995). The efficacy of psychosocial treatments in primary care: A review of randomized clinical trials. *General Hospital Psychiatry, 17*(6), 414–424.

Collins, C., Hewson, D. L., Munger, R., & Wade, T. (2010). *Evolving models of behavioral health integration into primary care*. New York: Milbank Memorial Fund.

Corso, K. A., Hunter, C. L., Dahl, O., Kallenberg, G. A., & Manson, L. (2016). *Integrating behavioral health into the medical home: A rapid implementation guide*. Phoenix, MD: Greenbranch Publishing.

Crain, L., Solberg, L., Unützer, J., Ohnsorg, K., Maciosek, M., Whitebird, R., et al. (2013). Designing and implementing research on a statewide quality improvement initiative: The DIAMOND study and initiative. *Medical Care, 51*, e58–e66. https://doi.org/10.1097/MLR.0b013e318249d8a4.

Cummings, N. A., Dorken, H., Pallak, M. S., & Henke, C. J. (1991). *The impact of psychological intervention on health care costs and utilization: The Hawaii Medicaid Project*. HCFA Contract Report #11-C-983344/9.

Cummings, N. A., & Follette, W. T. (1968). Psychiatric services and medical utilization in a prepaid health plan setting: Part 2. *Medical Care, 6*, 31–41.

deGruy, F., Dickinson, W., & Staton (2002). *20 Common Problems in Behavioral Health*. New York, NY: McGraw-Hill.

Depression Guideline Panel (1993). *Depression in Primary Care; Vol 2. Treatment of Major Depression*. (Clinical Practice Guideline No. 5, AHCPR Publication No. 93-0551). Rockville, MD: Department of Health and Human Services, Public Health Service, Agency for Health Care Policy and Research.

Engel, G. (1977). The need for a new medical model: a challenge for biomedicine. *Science 196* (4286), 129–136.

Fava, G. A., & Sonino, N. (2008). The biopsychosocial model thirty years later. *Psychotherapy and Psychosomatics, 77*, 1–2.

Follette, W. T., & Cummings, N. A. (1967). Psychiatric services and medical utilization in a prepaid health plan setting. *Medical Care, 5*(1), 25–35.

Freeman, D. (2011). The behavioral health medical home. In N. A. Cummings & W. T. O'Donohue (Eds.), *Understanding the behavioral healthcare crisis: The promise of integrated care and diagnostic reform* (pp. 250–265). Florence, KY: Routledge.

Gatchel, R. J., & Oordt, M. S. (2003). *Clinical health psychology and primary care: Practical advice and clinical guidance for successful collaboration*. Washington, DC: American Psychological Association.

Gerrity, M. (2016). *Evolving models of behavioral health integration: Evidence update 2010–2015*. New York: Milbank Memorial Fund.

Hall, J., Cohen, D. J., Davis, M., Gunn, R., Blount, A., Pollack, D. A., et al. (2015). Preparing the workforce for behavioral health and primary care integration. *Journal of the American Board of Family Medicine, 28*, S41–S51.

Hoge, M. A., Morris, J. A., Pomerantz, A., & Farley, T. (2014). *Core competencies for integrated behavioral health and primary care*. Washington, DC: SAMHSA-HRSA Center for Integrated Health Solutions.

Hunter, C. L., Goodie, J. L., Dobmeyer, A. C., Dorrance, K. A., & Anderson, N. B. (2014). Tipping points in the Department of Defense's experience with psychologists in primary care. *American Psychologist, 69*(4), 388–398.

Hunter, C. L., Goodie, J. L., Oordt, M., & Dobmeyer, A. C. (2009). *Integrated behavioral health in primary care: Step-by-step guidance for assessment and intervention*. Washington, DC: American Psychological Association.

Hunter, C. L., Goodie, J. L., Oordt, M., & Dobmeyer, A. C. (2017). *Integrated behavioral health in primary care: Step-by-step guidance for assessment and intervention* (2nd ed.). Washington, DC: American Psychological Association.

Institute for Clinical Systems Improvement. (2014). *The DIAMOND program: Treatment for patients with depression in primary care*. Retrieved from https://www.icsi.org/_asset/rs2qfi/DIAMONDWP0614.pdf

Institute of Medicine. (1996). *Primary care: America's health in a new era*. Washington DC: National Academy Press.

James, L. & O'Donohue, W. (2009). *The Primary Care Toolkit: Practical Resources for the Integrated Behavioral Care Provider*. New York, NY: Springer.

Kathol, R. G., DeGruy, F., & Rollman, B. L. (2014). Value-based financially sustainable behavioral health components in patient-centered medical homes. *Annals of Family Medicine, 12*(2), 172–175.

Katon, W., Robinson, P., Von Korff, M., Lin, E., Bush, T., Ludman, E., et al. (1996). A multifaceted intervention to improve treatment of depression in primary care. *Archives of General Psychiatry, 53*, 924–932.

Katon, W., & Schulberg, H. (1992). Epidemiology of depression in primary care. *General Hospital Psychiatry, 14*, 237–247.

Katon, W., Von Korff, M., Lin, E., Walker, E., Simon, G. E., Bush, T., et al. (1995). Collaborative management to achieve treatment guidelines. Impact on depression in primary care. *JAMA, 273*, 1026–1031.

Katon, W. J., Schoenbaum, M., Fan, M. Y., Callahan, C. M., Williams, J., Hunkeler, E., et al. (2005). Cost-effectiveness of improving primary care treatment of late-life depression. *Archives of General Psychiatry, 62*(12), 1313–1320.

Katon, W. J., Unutzer, J., Wells, K., & Jones, J. (2010). Collaborative depression care: History, evolution and ways to enhance dissemination and sustainability. *General Hospital Psychiatry, 32–35*, 456–464.

Keller, M., & Lavori, I. (1988). The adequacy of treating depression. *Journal of Nervous and Mental Disease, 176*, 471–474.

Kessler, R. (2015). Evaluating the process of mental health and primary care integration: The Vermont integration profile. *Family Medicine and Community Health, 3*, 63–65.

Kessler, R. C., McGonagle, K. A., Zhao, S., Nelson, C. B., Hughes, M., Eshleman, S., et al. (1994). Lifetime and 12-month prevalence of DSM- III–R psychiatric disorders in the United States. *Archives of General Psychiatry, 51*, 8–19.

Kroenke, K., & Mangelsdorff, A. D. (1989). Common symptoms in ambulatory care: Incidence, evaluation, therapy and outomces. *American Journal of Medicine, 86*, 262–266. New York, NY: W. W. Norton & Company, Inc.

Laygo, R., O'Donohue, W., Hall, S., Kaplan, A., Wood, R., Cummings, J., et al. (2003). Preliminary results from the Hawaii integrated healthcare project II. In N. A. Cummings, W. T. O'Donohue, & K. E. Ferguson (Eds.), *Behavioral health as primary care: Beyond efficacy to effectiveness* (pp. 111–144). Reno, NV: Context Press.

Macchi, C. R., Kessler, R., Auxier, A., Juvena, R., & Mullin, D. (2016). The practice integration profile: Rationale, development, method, and research. *Families, Systems & Health, 34*(4), 334–341.

Mark, T. L., Levit, K. R., & Buck, J. A. (2009). Datapoints: Psychotropic drug prescriptions by medical specialty. *Psychiatric Services, 60*(9), 1167.

McDaniel, S. H., Grus, C. L., Cubic, B. A., Hunter, C. L., Kearney, L. K., Schuman, C. C., et al. (2014). Competencies for psychology practice in primary care. *American Psychologist, 69*, 404–429.

Miller, B. F., Gilchrist, E. C., Ross, K. M., Wong, S. L., Blount, A., & Peek, C. J. (2016, February). *Core competencies for behavioral health providers working in primary care.* Prepared from the Colorado Consensus Conference.

Mynors-Wallis, L. M., Gath, D. H., Lloyd-Thomas, A. R., & Tomlinson, D. (1995). Randomized controlled trial comparing problem solving treatment with amitriptyline and placebo for major depression in primary care. *BMJ, 310*, 441–446.

Peek, C. J., Cohen, D. J., & deGruy, F. V. (2014). Research and evaluation in the transformation of primary care. *American Psychologist, 26*, 430–442.

Peek, C. J., & The National Integration Academy Council. (2013). *Lexicon for behavioral health and primary care integration: Concepts and definitions developed by expert consensus.* Rockville, MD: Agency for Healthcare Research and Quality.

Pratt, L.A., Brody, D.J., & Gu, Q. (2011). *Antidepressant use in persons aged 12 and over: United States, 2005–2008.* https://www.cdc.gov/nchs/data/databriefs/db76.htm. Hyattsville, MD: National Center for Health Statistics. Accessed 11 June 2017.

Regier, D. A., Myers, J. K., Kramer, M., Robins, L. N., Blazer, D. G., Hough, R. L., et al. (1984). The NIMH epidemiological catchment area program. Historical context, major objectives and study population characteristics. *Archives of General Psychiatry, 41*(10), 934–941.

Regier, D. A., Narrow, W. E., Rae, D. S., Manderscheid, R.W., Locke, B.Z. & Goodwin, F.K. (1993). The de facto US mental and addictive disorders service system: Epidemiologic catchment area and prospective 1-year prevalence rates of disorders and services. *Archives of General Psychiatry, 50*(2), 85–94.

Reiter, J., Dobmeyer, A., & Hunter, C. (2018). The Primary Care Behavioral Health (PCBH) model: An overview and operational definition. *Journal of Clinical Psychology in Medical Settings, 25*, 109–26.

Robinson, P. J., & Reiter, J. T. (2007). *Behavioral consultation and primary care: A guide to integrating services*. New York: Springer Science + Business Media.

Robinson, P. J., & Reiter, J. T. (2016). *Behavioral consultation and primary care: A guide to integrating services* (2nd ed.). Geneva, Switzerland: Springer International Publishing.

Schulberg, H. C., Coulehan, J. L., Block, M. R., Lave, J., Rodriquez, E., Scott, C. P., et al. (1993). Clinical trials of primary care treatment for major depression: Issues in design, recruitment and treatment. *International Journal of Psychiatry in Medicine, 23*, 29–42.

Serrano, N. (2015). *The implementer's guide to primary care behavioral health*. Available from https://itunes.apple.com/us/book/implementers-guide-to-primary/id833906873?mt=11

Serrano, N., Cordes, C., Cubic, B., & Daub, S. (2018). The State and Future of the Primary Care Behavioral Health Model of Service Delivery Workforce. *Journal of Clinical Psychology in Medical Settings 25*(2), 157–168.

Smith, R. C., Fortin, A. H., Dwamena, F., & Frankel, R. M. (2013). An evidence-based patient-centered method makes the biopsychosocial model scientific. *Patient Education and Counseling, 91*, 265–270.

Solberg, L. I., Crain, A. L., Jaeckels, N., Ohnsorg, K. A., Margolis, K. I., Beck, A., et al. (2013). The DIAMOND initiative: Implementing collaborative care for depression in 75 primary care clinics. *Implementation Science, 8*(135). https://doi.org/10.1186/1748-5908-8-135.

Strosahl, K. (1996). Primary mental health care: A new paradigm for achieving health and behavioral health integration. *Behavioral Healthcare Tomorrow, 5*, 93–96.

Strosahl, K. (1997). Building primary care behavioral health systems that work: A compass and a horizon. In N. Cummings, J. Cummings, & J. Johnson (Eds.), *Behavioral health in primary care: A guide for clinical integration* (pp. 37–68). Madison, CN: Psychosocial Press.

Strosahl, K. (1998). Integrating behavioral health and primary care services: The primary mental health care model. In A. Blount (Ed.), *Integrated primary care: The future of medical and mental health collaboration* (pp. 139–166). New York: Norton.

Strosahl, K. (2005). Training behavioral health and primary care providers for integrated care: A core competency approach. In W. T. O'Donohue, M. R. Byrd, N. A. Cummings, & D. A. Henderson (Eds.), *Behavioral integrative care: Treatments that work in primary care settings* (pp. 15–52). New York: Brunner-Routledge.

Unutzer, J. (2016). All hands-on deck. *Psychiatric News*. Retrieved from http://psychnews.psychiatryonline.org/doi/full/10.1176/appi.pn.2016.3a28

Unutzer, J., Katon, W., Callahan, C. M., Williams, J. W., Hunkeler, E., Harpole, L., et al. (2002). Collaborative care management of late-life depression in the primary care setting. *JAMA, 288*(22), 2836–2845.

U.S. Department of Education, Office of Planning, Evaluation, and Policy Development. (2010). *Evaluation of evidence-based practices in online learning: A meta-analysis and review of online learning studies*. Washington, DC: Author.

van Eeghen C, Kessler R, Littenberg B. (2017). Integrating Behavioral Health and Primary Care: A Toolkit. Burlington, Vermont.

Wagner, E. H., Austin, B. T., Davis, M., Hindmarsh, J., Schaefer, A., & Bonomi. (2001). Improving chronic illness care: Translating evidence into action. *Health Affairs, 20*(6), 64–78.

Wagner, E. H., Austin, B. T., & Von Korff, M. (1996). Organizing care for patients with chronic illness. *Milbank Quarterly, 74*(4), 511–544.

Wetzler, H. P., & Cruess, D. F. (1985). Self-reported physical health practices and health care utilization: Findings from the National Health Interview Survey. *American Journal of Public Health, 75*, 1329–1330.

Yano, E. M., Bair, M. J., Carrasquillo, O., Krein, S. L., & Rubenstein, L. V. (2014). Patient Aligned Care Teams (PACT): VA's journey to implementing patient-centered medical homes. *Journal of General Internal Medicine, 29*, 547–549.

Chapter 3
Enhancing Team-Based Skills in Primary Care: A Competency-Based Approach to Training and Workforce Development

C. R. Macchi and Rodger Kessler

Learning Objectives of This Chapter

Learners will:

1. Identify the interprofessional skills needed to operate effectively in an integrated team-based care environment.
2. Identify common behavioral health skill set shared among the professionals on an interprofessional medical team.
3. Analyze the training implications of the three worlds of healthcare practice on team-based care.
4. Apply the key dimensions of learning and instructional frameworks to develop a team-based practice curriculum.

Common Team-Based Practice Skill Set

Team-based care involves members each operating with a distinct set of skills that are related to their training and experience. Performing effectively and efficiently as a team requires each team member to develop an additional, complimentary skill set. These shared core competencies facilitate the effective delivery of integrated healthcare. George Thibault, M.D., president of the Josiah Macy Jr. Foundation, stated in a conference report,

C. R. Macchi (✉) · R. Kessler
Integrated Behavioral Health Programs, College of Health Solutions,
Arizona State University, Phoenix, AZ, USA
e-mail: crmacchi@asu.edu; Rodger.Kessler@asu.edu

C. R. Macchi, R. Kessler (eds.), *Training to Deliver Integrated Care*,
https://doi.org/10.1007/978-3-319-78850-0_3

> The health care system will not be able to keep pace with these explosive changes unless it moves to a team-based care model. But the delivery system cannot make that shift effectively until the education system begins to train new health professionals in collaborative practice. (Josiah Macy Jr. Foundation & Interprofessional Education Collaborative, 2011, p. 9)

This chapter reviews the latest initiatives to identify common, team-based specialized skills. We aim to challenge the current view that assumes behavioral health-related core competencies as associated with a *specific role* (i.e., Behavioral Health Practitioner (BHP)) and instead focus on the BH *function* that is incorporated, at varying levels, within the scope of each team member's practice (C. Hunter & Goodie, 2010). We propose specific training strategies and approaches that are designed to support learner development of team-based core competencies that integrate medical and behavioral care throughout the continuum of whole-person care. The Interprofessional Education Collaborative (IPEC) provides a set of core competencies focused on team-based care including values and ethics, roles and responsibilities for collaborative practice, interprofessional communication, and teamwork and team-based care (Interprofessional Education Collaborative Expert Panel, 2011). While a multitude of core competency lists and descriptions have been proposed, currently they lack guidance to operationalize and assess member skill development. This chapter addresses that gap by providing pedagogical recommendations for effective training approaches targeting specific team-based skills intended to improve patient outcomes (Havyer et al., 2013; Mitchell et al., 2012).

Multiple Dimensions of a Team-Based Approach to Integrated Healthcare

A team-based approach reflects a simultaneous engagement of several dimensions of care delivery including individual roles, shared responsibilities, and ongoing participation (see Fig. 3.2). Each team member contributes unique expertise and experiences to the process of care, while each contribution to the comprehensive care plan is complimentary to the others (i.e., individual domains). The members' focus on shared goals, contributions to treatment planning, and continuous communication and adaptation to patient changes facilitates comprehensive care delivery (i.e., overlapping domains). The participation of each member supports the patient's engagement in effective self-management (i.e., patient at center of the team). Each dimension of team-based care is facilitated by a set of core competencies that require training and refinement (Fig. 3.1).

Team Members' Roles: Overlapping and Complimentary Each team member's overlapping role entails specific skills and duties that require particular training and expertise to expand the member's scope of practice. A patient-centered team consistently addresses two overarching questions related to complimentary roles: (1) Which team members can best address the patient need? And (2) what combination of team member involvement would most effectively and efficiently address that

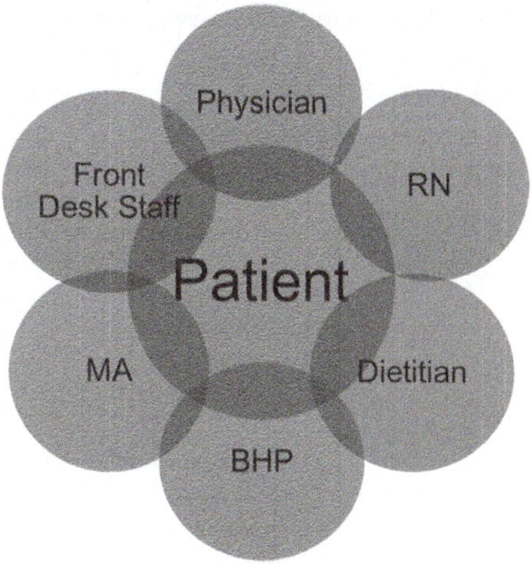

Fig. 3.1 Dimensions of team-based care – roles, responsibilities, and participation

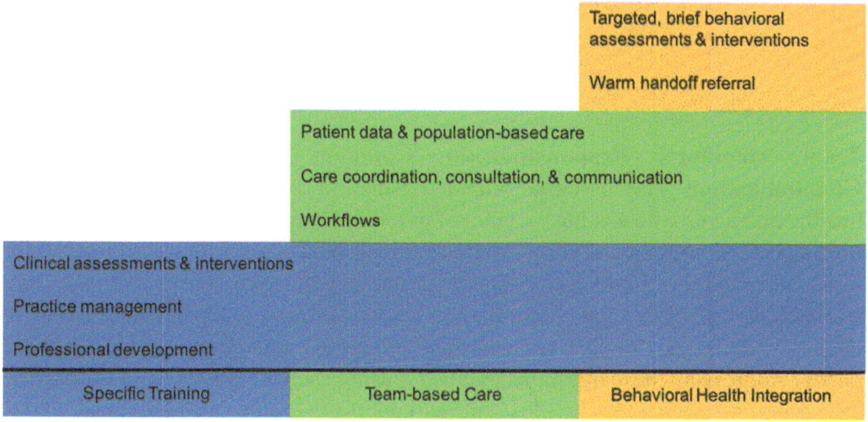

Fig. 3.2 Example of layered competencies

need? A physician, trained to focus primarily on the patients' physical health conditions, looks beyond that scope of practice to identify the other related behavioral dimensions of the patients' conditions. Operating within a medical team where awareness, trust, and ongoing collaboration among the members have evolved, the physician becomes better prepared to identify overlaps and gaps in personal training and experience. Additional training that builds upon the physician's foundational medical training and experience focuses on team-based approaches that address medical-behavioral comorbidities (see Fig. 3.2). In this example, the physician becomes increasingly aware of the potential for expanding one's scope of practice while simultaneously identifying the limitations of that role. Experiencing this tension provides the physician with repeated opportunities to actively collaborate with the other team members and identify their shared responsibilities.

Table 3.1 Integrated team-based approach: common objectives, involvement, and outcomes

Area of focus	Team-based objectives	Practitioner involvement	Outcomes
Patient care and support	• Chronic care management • Patient self-management • Population health-focused • Prevention-focused • Whole-person care	• Eliciting patient input and patient interactions • Patient monitoring • Patient responsiveness • Population health management	• Engaged patients • Expanded access to team services • Improved patient health outcomes • Increased patient satisfaction • Increased patient self-management
Team performance	• Communication • Community engagement • Shared goals • Shared records • Shared treatment plan	• Clear and complementary roles • Maximizing expertise • Operating at top of license • Shared responsibilities • Trust among team members	• Decreased healthcare costs • Facilitative system transformation • Increased team cohesiveness • Improved team efficiencies

Team Member's Responsibilities: Common Goals, Planning, and Communication The essential characteristics of a team-based approach to healthcare begins with a cohesive team of practitioners who are focused on common objectives and subsequent efforts that are aimed at accomplishing specific, multi-level outcomes (see Table 3.1). A patient-centered team consistently addresses two overarching questions related to common responsibilities: (1) What are the patient needs? And (2) how can each team member effectively and efficiently address those needs? Addressing these questions entails focusing each member's skills and expertise on common objectives while coordinating efforts to improve outcomes.

A team-based approach simultaneously focuses on two areas of responsibility: patient care and support while monitoring and adjusting team performance. Shared team responsibilities establish common team objectives, specify practitioner involvement with patients and other team members, and monitor patient outcomes and team performance metrics. While individual members have varied roles, they support the common functions that are effective for reaching the maximum number of patients within multiple populations of need. Effective teams coherently integrate patient medical and behavioral monitoring, assessments, interventions, and follow-ups.

Team Member's Participation: Patient Engagement Team-based care that focuses exclusively on patient populations has the potential to dehumanize individual patients and depersonalize their experience of receiving care. A "one-size-fits-all" approach to individual patients within a particular patient population should be replaced with an approach that matches the unique characteristics of each patient with a tailored approach to care. A patient-centered team consistently addresses three overarching questions related to patient engagement: (1) Which of the patient's strengths and resources can be utilized to address the patient's need? (2) How can that patient participate as an integral team member to effectively and efficiently address that need? And (3) how does the system of care support the activated patient within the team? Examination of a team-based approach from the patient's perspective highlights multiple dimensions of patient engagement in team-based care. The experience of a patient receiving the appropriate treatment at the right time would encounter a team that supports the knowledge, skills, and motivation to engage in health behavior changes needed for sustainable self-management.

The Three Worlds and Interprofessional Core Competencies

Effective integrated team-based healthcare begins with the assumption that all of the members of a team share a common set of core competencies and workforce development programs should address those common traits (Hoge, Tondora, & Marrell, 2005). Team members have a set of skills needed to effectively address each of the three interdependent worlds or dimensions of the practice (C. Hunter & Goodie, 2010; Peek, 2008). Peek (2008) identified three interdependent dimensions (i.e., clinical, operational, financial) of healthcare practice in real-world settings (see Fig. 3.3). These three dimensions relate to performance expectations at each level and among professionals within a healthcare practice (i.e. practice, manager, practitioner, interprofessional). The interdependent nature of these dimensions applies to the individual professionals and interprofessional collaborations in integrated healthcare practices. A professional primarily responsible for addressing one dimension (e.g., BHP providing clinical services) is required to simultaneously be aware of and incorporate practices related to the other two dimensions. This simultaneous engagement is necessary to provide effective, sustainable programs and services. In other words, effective clinical services are inextricably related to the operational systems and financial management occurring within the practice. Effective training programs must equip learners with the ability to understand and operate among these three interconnected dimensions of healthcare practice.

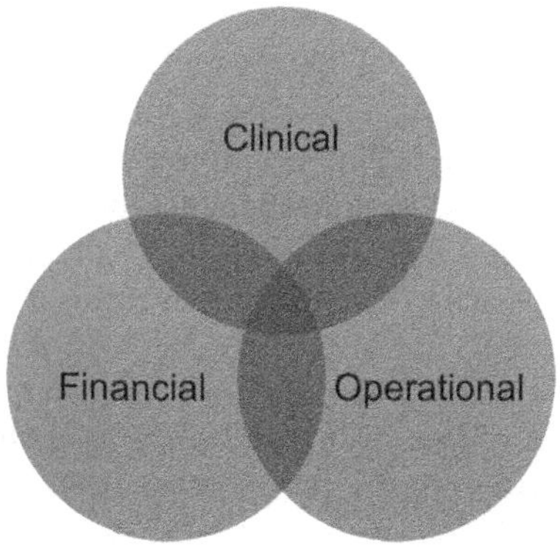

Fig. 3.3 Dimensions of healthcare practice – clinical, operational, financial

Several initiatives have resulted in reports of the work of teams tasked with identifying a common set of core competencies for behavioral health in primary care. The Interprofessional Education Collaborative (IPEC, 2011), American Psychological Association (APA, 2013), Substance and Mental Health Services Administration and Health Resources and Services Administration (SAMHSA and HRSA, 2015), Agency for Healthcare Research and Quality (AHRQ) (Kinman, Gilchrist, Payne-Murphy, & Miller, 2015), and Eugene S. Farley Jr. Health Policy Center (2016) each published detailed literature reviews of provider- and staff-level competencies. In this chapter we are adopting the proposed definition of provider and staff competencies described as "the knowledge, skills, and attitudes that allow an individual to perform tasks and roles in an integrated primary care setting" (AHRQ, 2015, p. 10). A crosswalk of the results of those five initiatives categorizes the proposed core competencies corresponding with each of the three world dimensions (see Table 3.2). These competencies provide the foundation for the unique skills that each member contributes to the work of the team. Note that none of the reports identify competencies that address the financial dimension of healthcare practice.

The training challenge remains as we have several lists of core competencies that address many of the same activities and related skills but provide no mechanism for measuring each provider competency level. Looking ahead, the next step toward identifying and operationalizing competencies would be to develop an instrument to measure current levels and provide a basis upon which to compare levels at varying points throughout a practitioner's developmental trajectory. Valid, reliable training evaluations are needed to standardize the training of medical teams addressing patients' BH issues. The usefulness of measures will depend largely on those that specify targeted performance metrics. The remainder of this chapter addresses ways to use the existing lists to guide training development, implementation, and evaluation of learner outcomes.

Training Objectives Designed to Address Three World Dimensions of Team-Based Practice

The work of Behavioral Health Practitioners (BHP) and Integrated Health Care (IHC) Managers requires a simultaneous engagement with the three worlds (i.e., clinical, operational, financial) of integrated healthcare delivery (Peek, 2008). The eventual identification of a common set of core competencies and associated performance metrics must address all three of these dimensions and the interdependence of each to the other. While the healthcare field lacks a clear consensus on integrated behavioral healthcare practices, a comparison of practices requires identifying a common set of key skills for each member of the care team. Identifying these skills is a prerequisite for comparing performance data and refining training approaches designed to accomplish the Triple Aim objectives.

Table 3.2 Crosswalk of core competencies on three world dimensions

Three world dimensions	IPEC (2011) *Core competencies for interprofessional collaborative practice*	APA Health Psychology (2013) *Competencies for psychology practice in PC*	AHRQ (2015) *Provider- and practice-level competencies for integrated BH in PC*	SAMHSA/HRSA (2015) *Core competencies for integrated BH and PC*	Eugene S. Farley Jr. (2016) *Competencies for BH providers working in PC*
Clinical		Assessment of BH risk factors	Identification and assessment of BH needs	Screening and assessment	Identify and assess BH needs as part of primary care team
		EVB interventions that encourage proper use of healthcare resources	Treatment of BH needs	Care planning and care coordination Intervention	
	Patient-centered care	Demonstrates awareness, sensitivity, and skills in working professionally with diverse individuals	Patient engagement Whole-person care and cultural competency	Care planning and care coordination Cultural competence and adaptation	Engage and activate patients in their care Provide efficient and effective care delivery that meets the needs of the population of the primary care setting
Operational		Planning and implementing organizational changes to optimize service delivery Practice management	Primary care culture: Agenda setting, prioritization, and strategizing provider workflow	Systems-oriented practice	Provide culturally responsive, whole-person and family-oriented care
	Coordinated effort across professions	Interprofessionalism Individual, cultural, and disciplinary diversity Building and sustaining relationships in PC	Team-based care and collaboration	Collaboration and teamwork	Work as a primary care team member to create and implement care plans that address BH factors

(continued)

Table 3.2 (continued)

Three world dimensions	IPEC (2011) *Core competencies for interprofessional collaborative practice*	APA Health Psychology (2013) *Competencies for psychology practice in PC*	AHRQ (2015) *Provider- and practice-level competencies for integrated BH in PC*	SAMHSA/HRSA (2015) *Core competencies for integrated BH and PC*	Eugene S. Farley Jr. (2016) *Competencies for BH providers working in PC*
	Teamwork communication	Clinical consultation	Communication	Interpersonal communication	Help observe and improve care team function and relationships Communicate effectively with other providers, staff, and patients
		Professional values and attitudes	Professional values and attitudes		Understand, value, and adapt to the diverse professional cultures of an integrated care team
	Continuous improvement efforts	Track patient outcomes and program evaluation		Practice-based learning and quality improvement	
	Informatics	Effective use of information technology		Informatics	
Financial	NA	NA	NA	NA	NA

Effective training programs must equip practitioners with the core competencies to engage simultaneously in each of the three worlds of healthcare delivery. Mastery of one world is dependent upon a keen responsiveness to the influences that the three worlds have on one another. Core competencies have traditionally focused on the unique cultures and skills of the siloed professions that they represent. Clinical training programs often place an emphasis on the development of assessment, intervention, and evaluation skills for delivering one aspect of whole-person care programs and services (e.g., medical, dietary, occupational, physical therapy, social work, or mental health). The evidence rarely reveals programs that train the learner to understand, engage in, and collaborate with the operational and financial systems that support the delivery of that care. Additionally, training should address the natural tensions and impacts among the three dimensions of healthcare delivery (i.e., clinical, operational, and financial). The interactions that occur among professional collaborations require each team member to develop a multidimensional skill set that involves translating cultural perspectives, establishing common goals, effective communication, negotiation strategies, and decision-making. Peek (2008) suggests that each professional must be equipped to "take a three world view" (p. 32) of the whole practice and each of its programs and services. Education and training introduces a fourth worldview that is addressed in this manual.

A training approach that addresses the evolving healthcare marketplace must incorporate strategies that address the emerging evidence for team-based care (Burgess, McGregor, & Mellis, 2014; Rosenman, Ilgen, Shandro, Harper, & Fernandez, 2015). Instructional approaches should not only provide learners with opportunities to obtain knowledge and refine skills needed today, those approaches must also explicitly provide the meta-skills needed to adjust and adapt to tomorrow's opportunities and challenges.

Guiding Principles for Integrated Team-Based Training and Workforce Development

Training programs that are designed to target adult professionals in practice settings at each phase employ a pedagogical approach that incorporates scaffolding, contextual learning, self-directed learning, and modeling (Merriam & Bierema, 2014). Lev Vygotsky (1978) introduced the concept of scaffolding to describe an incremental, step-by-step instruction process that engages learners at the boundaries of their current competency level. Existing knowledge and experiences become the platform upon which the learner is instructed and incorporates new information or skills. Contextual learning consistently addresses the relevance of that new knowledge and the application of the new skills. The science of integrated medicine and behavioral health is continuously evolving. Effective training programs must be designed to equip practitioners to learn new knowledge and skills through self-directed, lifelong learning that equips the learner to be responsive to and adapt to those changes

(Hoge, Huey, & O'Connell, 2004). Modeling occurs in environments where learners observe and engage with other colleagues at varying levels of competence (i.e., field placements, residencies, internships, and fellowships). Practitioners engaging in these interprofessional experiences have repeated opportunities to discover, apply, and further refine clinical- and team-based skills.

One way to conceptualize a team-based training program is to identify a list of principles then design learning modules that address the related topics. Addressing dynamic team development and productivity requires an approach that can adequately address both team characteristics and processes. We are proposing the use of a time-related framework that separates training principles, content, and team-based activities into the following time phases (see Fig. 3.4): (1) preparation, (2) implementation, and (3) evaluation.

Learners who have limited or no team-based experience may benefit from beginning with the preparation phase. These early phase training programs are often associated with graduate degrees, employee orientation modules, or practices with little or no team-based experience. Educational training programs offered to existing teams that are currently engaged in ongoing and continuous practice may target any phase in the framework. Preparation phase curriculum is intended to expose the

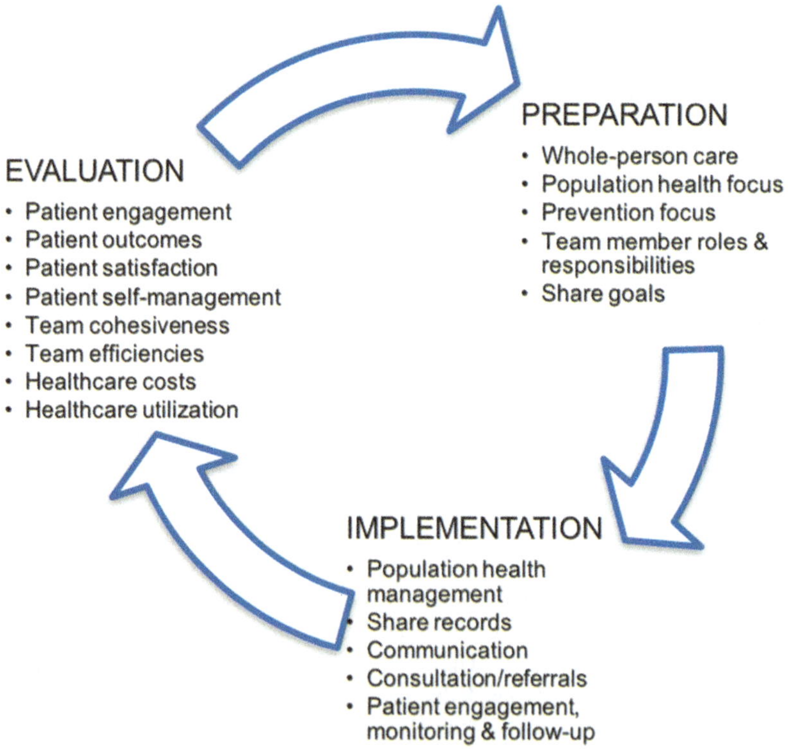

Fig. 3.4 Training phases

learner to foundational integrated team-based concepts and strategies needed to effectively perform on integrated care teams. Curriculum targeting the implementation phase addresses topics related to clinical- and team-related performance activities. Evaluation phase curriculum addresses topics related to patient- and team-related performance outcomes and the mechanisms that facilitate ongoing quality improvement processes. Though each training phase addresses distinct objectives and activities, the combination of the three phases provides a developmental, iterative framework that addresses the interconnected nature of the phases and their associations with patient engagement, team processes, and patient and team outcomes.

Team Preparation Training Phase Training at this early phase addresses the foundational principles of whole-person, team-based care (see Table 3.3). The training equips team members to conceptualize individual patients' health issues using a biopsychosocial lens while organizing the team to identify and address population health management and early intervention, prevention-focused efforts. The combined effect of these concepts is intended to maximize the team's efforts and use of available resources to produce the maximum results. This phase begins with the assumption that each practitioner has a level of training and experience in their specific profession. Building upon this assumption, the training also addresses the ways to actively engage patients as part of the care team that is focused on shared goals, responsibilities, and functions. The members are trained to set common patient health outcome targets that guide assessment and intervention choices.

Team Implementation Training Phase Second phase training builds upon the foundational principles established in the preparation phase. Implementation training provides learners with the specific, measureable skills and practices that are needed to effectively operate on a care team. The team is trained to conceptually step back from a focus on individual patients to identify patterns and trends of health conditions and comorbidities among groups of comparable patients. The team, using this population health management approach, begins by reviewing the

Table 3.3 Early phase training objectives: foundations of team development and team-based care

	View of patient	View of team
Whole-person care	Biopsychosocial approach to care	Integrated medical and behavioral patient visits
Population health focus	Identify and monitor of patient populations	Magnify team efforts to reach more patients
Prevention focus	Engaged in early interventions to limit emergence of comorbidities	Identify reallocation of team resources toward early interventions
Roles and responsibilities	Focused on patient engagement	Shared team member functions
Shared goals	Shared improved health outcome targets	Focused on supporting other team members' efforts

Table 3.4 The Five As model: a guide for a team-based approach

Phases	Key objectives
Assess	Determine health issues related to patient's current symptoms and functioning
Advise	Summarize health issues and provide behavior change options
Agree	Determine what the patient is interested in doing
Assist	Address new behavioral skills, problem-solving skills, and barriers to change
Arrange	Follow-up plan and/or referrals

health records or surveying patients during routine visits to determine those who may benefit from standardized clinical pathways and protocols. Members are trained to communicate and consult with one another in a fashion that support the other member's efforts. Additionally, shared, common medical records further support asynchronous communication and reinforce shared treatment plans. The Five As (i.e., assess, advise, agree, assist, arrange) (C. L. Hunter, Goodie, Oordt, & Dobmeyer, 2009) provides a useful framework to guide each practitioner as they engage with patients within the scope of their specific role on the team. The patient's experience with each member using this common framework reinforces the integrated approach to patient involvement, common health issue conceptualizations, planning, steps toward improving health outcomes, and follow-up or referral recommendations. Team-based implementation training provides specific strategies and techniques for each step in this treatment process. Using a stepped-care approach, the team continually assesses the patient to determine if advancing the care and referring to a team member are needed to provide a more intensive level of treatment (Table 3.4).

Team Evaluation Training Phase Assessment of the team functioning and the patient experience is the final phase of training. This evaluation phase trains the team to consider three groups of outcomes each reflecting the effects of the integrated team-based efforts including patient health-related outcomes, team performance outcomes, and healthcare costs and utilization outcomes. Teams are trained to understand and interpret performance metrics for each group and consider alternative healthcare management strategies that may produce even better results.

Teams learn to identify patient engagement, health outcomes, satisfaction, and self-management improvements signaling the degree to which patients are playing an active role on the care team and adjusting health behaviors to more effectively manage health conditions.

The teams are provided with the opportunity to examine the performance of the team as a whole. This training provides team members with the skills to assess the level of team cohesiveness and improved efficiencies that allow them to maximize the time spent with patients and the use of available resources. Improved team efficiencies have the potential of increasing the team's access to more patients. An example of a Behavioral Health Practitioner (BHP) performance scale illustrates specific items that are focused on the core competencies associated with each of the three worlds (i.e., clinical, operational, financial) (see Appendix). This assessment specifies specific within broader domains of activities, observed care behavioral anchors, and potential situations where the evaluator is directed to observe those behaviors. Finally, the team is trained to monitor and interpret additional metrics related to healthcare costs and utilization rates to determine potential savings and decreasing patient need of services.

Interconnected Training Phases The interconnected nature of each phase and their relationships to patient engagement, team processes, and patient and team outcomes points to a useful feedback mechanism for repeated training and practice refinements. Team learning and resulting adjustments in one phase provide opportunities and information to be processed in another phase of training. An example is when teams have the outcomes data from the evaluation phase, this data can provide information to reexamine the foundational structures of the team when repeating phase one training. This quality improvement strategy suggests that the iterative process of the three phases is ongoing and continuous. Effective training programs should engage in each phase of training while incorporating opportunities to revisit the elements of the other phases.

Steps Toward Developing an Effective Training Program

We have discussed the guiding principles for developing integrated, team-based care training programs. These principles provide the conceptual framework needed to determine the overall structure of a training program. In this section, we address examples of specific learning objectives, training activities, and performance assessment strategies needed to develop, implement, and evaluate the effects of an effective, competence-based training program (see Table 3.5).

A compass is a useful tool that indicates the direction of a traveler's journey; however, without a map, the traveler may simply wander and potentially get lost.

Learning Objectives, Training Activities, and Performance Assessments The development of an effective training course begins with identifying targeted, measureable learning objectives. The examples of the learning objectives illustrate specific ways to address each training topic (see Table 3.5). The topics are conceptual

Table 3.5 Integrated team-based training development plan

		Examples		
Training phase	Topics	Learning objectives	Training activities	Performance assessments
Preparation	• Whole-person care	• Translate biopsychosocial model into primary care context	• Review relevant literature	• 5-min presentation that includes key issues
	• Population health focus	• Distinguish between the individual patient- and population-focused model of care	• Create a graphic illustrating the differences between the two	• Completed graphic of distinctions
	• Prevention focus	• Analyze the life course of disease and the potential effects of earlier intervention	• Develop two different primary care prevention pathways	• Discuss the similarities and differences between the prevention pathways
	• Roles and responsibilities	• Define and operationalize team care and roles within the primary care team	• Identify a common primary care problem; list the members of the team and identify their roles; develop a shared care plan and identify the medical-behavioral and patient contributions	• Review an example of successful team-based care
	• Shared goals	• Identify the medical and behavioral elements of frequently seen medical issues; identify the core elements of a population health model and examples of potential outcomes	• Develop a population-based algorithm to be established in a primary care practice	• Review the algorithm with a practice physician and practice manager
Implementation	• Population health management	• Examine populations of patients with specific health conditions and care needs	• Analyze a practice data set identifying patient subpopulations	• Describe distinct features of each subpopulation
	• Shared records	• Define the issues involved in generating shared records	• Review available literature	• Successfully increase the elements and flow of a shared record
	• Communication	• Identify methods of shared communication	• Interview members of disciplines other than one's own about core communication issues in patient care	• Discuss clinical examples of shared communication
	• Consultation/ referrals	• Demonstrate the core skills of consultation in primary care	• Role-play different consultation scenarios	• Discuss the new learning form of the role-play
	• Patient engagement, monitoring, and follow-up	• Discuss current state of patient engagement and list different methods to improve the process	• Interview a patient(s) about what is important to them in order to be engaged in their care	• Present how current thinking and practice would change based on patient feedback

Evaluation	• Patient engagement	• Identify the ratio of those initiating treatment to the percentage of patients involved in care plan generation	• Collect data about referrals vs. attended appointment	• Propose changes designed to enhance patient treatment initiation
	• Patient outcomes	• Review methods of generating and using outcome and satisfaction data	• Review available EHR data to identify available outcome measures; complete at least three clinical outcome measures	• Suggest a core set of measures and methods to regularly collect patient outcomes
	• Patient satisfaction	• Identify key dimensions of patient satisfaction related to involvement with care team treatment plan development and decision-making	• Administer patient survey	• Identify care team process modifications based upon data analysis
	• Patient self-management	• Apply different models and measures to support patient engagement in their care	• Review literature of patient self-management strategies	• Propose an integrated set of patient self-management strategies
	• Team cohesiveness	• Explore a care team's shared goals, responsibilities, and referral practices	• Interview then compare the members' perceptions of a care team	• Critical analysis of team members'
	• Team efficiencies	• Review three different methods of care improvement used in primary care	• Create a dummy quality improvement project	• Review project with other clinician and generate their feedback
	• Healthcare costs	• List the elements of total healthcare costs and how to compute it	• Collect published estimates of costs associated with BH comorbidities	• Successfully calculate expected total costs with an integrated method
	• Healthcare utilization	• Identify all sources of healthcare utilization	• Identify drivers of excessive utilization	• Identify three strategies that have successfully impacted utilization

Table 3.6 Example assignment assessment rubric

Criterion	Unacceptable	Acceptable	Good	Excellent
Description of biopsychosocial model in primary care	Missing or unclear description of the model (0 points)	Description of the model lacks a relationship to primary care; exclusively uses personal observation to support the thesis of the presentation (1 point)	Description of both the model and its relationship to primary care is vaguely connected; includes less than three references to support the thesis of the presentation (1.5 points)	Description of both the model and its relationship to primary care is clearly connected and succinct; includes three or more references to support the thesis of the presentation (2.5 points)

constructs associated with integrated team-based care. Development of a learning objective provides a statement that describes the intended results of the learner's engagement in the training process that is focused on that topic. The approach to addressing that topic could result in varied learning activities depending upon the trainer's conceptualization or point of view.

Consider the first topic of whole-person care. The meaning of this topic may seem evident to most; however, training may take several different approaches. Whole-person care could be described in each of the following ways: a treatment approach addressing the multiple dimensions of a patient's illness; an educational approach that addresses a patient's convergent and divergent roles in varied settings; or, as suggested, an approach that addresses the treatment of the biological, psychological, and social (biopsychosocial) dimensions of health behaviors and chronic condition management specifically occurring in a primary care setting. Once the objective is determined, the training activity can be designed to assist the learner through a process of reviewing the multiple applications of the biopsychosocial model. The use of the model in primary care, as compared and contrasted with other settings, is intended to highlight the unique application. Finally, to determine the effect of the training on the learner's comprehension and application of the model, the program requires the learner to present the results of the learning, thus providing the trainer with an opportunity to observe and assess the learner's performance. An effective assessment is developed when the trainer anticipates and describes the learner's demonstration of specific, measureable skills. Assessment rubrics are often developed to detail the varying levels of performance on multiple dimensions (see Table 3.6).

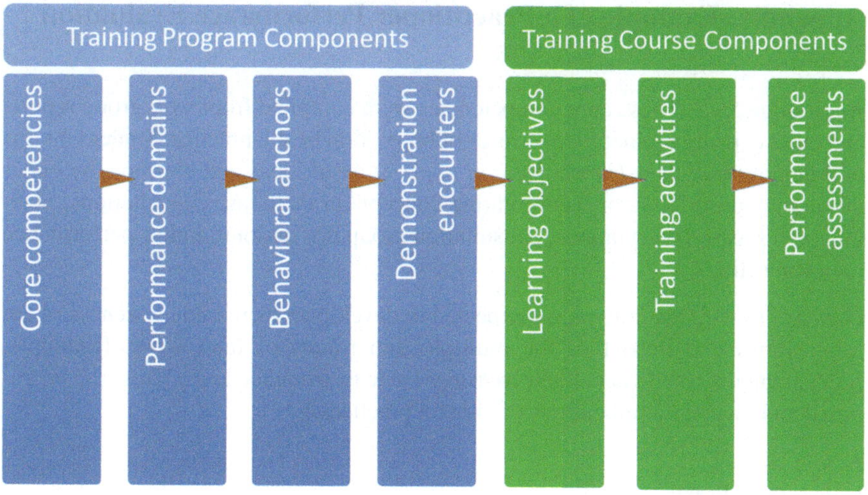

Fig. 3.5 Linked program and course components

Training Program Development and Performance Evaluation The previous section addressed the elements of a training course. A comprehensive training program that is comprised of a collection of individual courses should have a set of overarching program core competencies and objectives. A program is then developed to link the overarching core competencies to the learning objectives within the individual courses (see Fig. 3.5). The expected outcomes of the overall program design inform the development of each course component.

The ongoing assessment of a learner's skill development is captured in systematic assessments targeting specific skills targeting the core competencies along the learning continuum (Havyer et al., 2013; Institute of Medicine, 2015; Robinson & Reiter, 2016; Stanhope, Solomon, Pernell-Arnold, Sands, & Bourjolly, 2005) (see Appendix – Example of a Practitioner Performance Evaluation for doctoral interns). The evaluation addresses multiple performance domains each related to the set of core competencies: conceptual and professional development, clinical skills/practice, practice management, collaboration, and four additional items related to the practitioner's attention to financial related to team-based practice. The learner's demonstrated use of the biopsychosocial framework in a course may also be assessed in practice using the behavioral anchors listed in lines 11 and 12 of that performance evaluation (see Appendix).

Appendix: Example of a Practitioner Performance Evaluation

Knowledge/Skill These core competencies were compiled from workgroup reports and other existing evaluation measures of behavioral health practice. Student interns will demonstrate their *knowledge and application* of ideas and concepts by either discussing, describing, or incorporating concepts in their case consultations, planning notes, case presentations, consultation group discussions, and/or performance review meetings.

Dimensions Student interns are expected to develop an increased awareness of the implications and impact of the multiple dimensions of their work. (Example: Student interns should become increasingly able to articulate and address the operational and financial implications of clinical practices.)

- C = clinical
- O = operational
- F = financial

Behavioral Anchors The behaviors that the evaluator may observe in the course of working with the student intern

Focus of Evaluation This column lists the most likely places that the student intern would demonstrate the behaviors that are to be evaluated.

Item evaluation scale (select ☒ the column that applies to each item)

- Proficient – The student intern *consistently demonstrates* behaviors that are appropriate and applicable to the current work.
- Progressing – The student intern *occasionally demonstrates* behaviors that are appropriate and applicable to the current work.
- Missing – The student intern *does not demonstrate* behaviors when it would be appropriate and applicable to the current work.
- Not observed – The student *has not had the opportunity* for the evaluator to observe the student's behavior.

	Knowledge or skill	Dimensions	Care behavioral anchors	Focus of evaluation	Proficient	Progressing	Missing	Not observed
Conceptual and professional development								
1	Systems orientation	C	Identifies clinical models that are appropriate for the primary care setting	Verbal report to mentor includes description of approach among range of models				
2		O	Identifies policies and procedures related to sustaining integrated practices	Refers to related on-site policies in descriptions of clinical practices				
3	Primary care culture	C	Communicates unique features of primary care setting	Suggests clinical approaches that work well within primary care setting				
4		O	Practices brief hallway consultations with other clinic providers	Review of occurrences of hallway handoffs				
5	Cultural adaptation	C	Readily available for warm handoffs during patient exam visits	Available to provide patients with immediate BH assistance				
6		O	Collaboration with medical team performance	Feedback from medical team reports about intern support of medical team goals				
7	Professionalism	C	Clearly describes the unique, complimentary roles of each member of the interprofessional medical team	Performs a unique clinical role on interprofessional medical team				
8		O	Collaborates well with other providers in the clinic	Medical team feedback about student intern collaborative interactions				

(continued)

	Knowledge or skill	Dimensions	Care behavioral anchors	Focus of evaluation	Proficient	Progressing	Missing	Not observed
9	Practice-based learning	C	Generates educational opportunities for practice members to examine behavioral factors related to patient medical conditions (e.g., lunch and learns)	Review list of presentations student intern shared with medical team				
10		O	Attends regular medical staff learning opportunities (e.g., grand rounds)	Review list of presentations attended				
11	Biopsychosocial orientation	C	Describes the behavioral, physical, and relational dimensions of patients' medical issues	Review feedback from medical team				
12		O	Supports integrated clinical pathways that provide comprehensive treatment of targeted patients	Review student intern's treatment plans				
13	Quality improvement	C	Identifies targets for behaviorally oriented, quality improvement projects	Proposes steps for a quality improvement plan				
14		O	Regularly participates in improvement conversations	Provides useful suggestions for improving clinical practice				

Clinical skills/practice								
15	Screening and assessment of behavioral health issues related to medical conditions	C	Consistently uses validated outcome measures to assess patients	Review list of measures used				
16		O	Translates assessment results in practical terms that support the work of the medical team	Summary note for medical team in patient medical record				
17	Population-based approaches	C	Identifies needs and approaches to address patient populations	Review student intern's use of population-based protocols				
18		O	Participates in care pathways that support medical team responses to patient population needs	Role of BH in care pathways				
19	Evidence-based interventions	C	Uses evidence-based interventions related to focused, patient populations	Review list of evidence-based approaches				
20		O	Chooses evidence-based interventions that support integrated pathways	Student intern reports identifying specific data fields from patient medical records or EHR				
21	Informatics and data	C	Engages in bi-directional, transparent notes and communication with other medical team members thru EHR	Review content and communications within student intern's clinical notes				
22		O	Uses template EHR for clinical notes	Review accuracy of student intern's clinical notes				

(continued)

	Knowledge or skill	Dimensions	Care behavioral anchors	Focus of evaluation	Proficient	Progressing	Missing	Not observed
Practice management								
23	Documentation	C	Develops clinical notes that provide a clear and succinct summary of patient BH issues directly related to medical condition(s)	Review clarity and form of student intern's clinical notes				
24		O	Develops clear, accurate EHR notes that are understandable and useful to other medical team members	Review applicability of student intern's clinical notes to other team members' roles				
25	Time management	C	Performs brief, targeted patient assessments and interventions	Student intern's visits with patients average less than 30 min				
26		O	Work with patients supports the established clinic workflow	Feedback from medical director and other medical team members of student intern's participation in workflows				
27	Resource management	C	Appropriately refers patients to self-management and/or community resources with clear rationale for referral	Review the relevance of the list of resources referred to patient conditions and needs				
28		O	Appropriately refers patients to other medical team members with clear rationale for referral	Feedback from medical team that intern provides appropriate referrals				

29	Compliance with clinic policies and protocols	C	Uses approaches to patient care that are consistent with clinic policies	Feedback from team lead that intern supports clinic policies and procedures				
30		O	Demonstrates support of existing clinic workflows and practices	Feedback from medical team that intern supports practices				
Collaboration								
31	Communication with providers and patients	C	Describes clear connections between patients' BH issues and their medical conditions	Feedback from medical team that intern clarifies relationship of BH issues to patient medical conditions				
32		O	Identifies ways collaborative care can effectively address patient medical and behavioral issues	Feedback from medical team that intern discusses team-based care efforts				
33	Interprofessional relationships	C	Consults with medical team members to support patient medical outcomes	Feedback from medical team that intern seeks out consultations				
34		O	Develops relationships to supports clinic practices	Feedback from medical team that intern discusses ways to coordinate practice				
35	Care coordination	C	Explores with patients ways to use the various medical team resources	Review description of referrals within student intern's clinical notes				
36		O	Provides accurate and sufficient information necessary for other team members to provide patient continuity of care	Review recommendations within student intern's clinical notes				

(continued)

	Knowledge or skill	Dimensions	Care behavioral anchors	Focus of evaluation	Proficient	Progressing	Missing	Not observed
37	Identifies and supports medical team shared goals	C	Communicates with patients about the medical team's treatment goals	Review relevance to treatment goals within student intern's clinical notes				
38		O	Addresses shared goals during case consultations and staff meetings	Connections of case review reports to shared medical team goals				
39	Supports patient engagement on care team	C	Invites patients to contribute to the treatment decision-making processes	Review descriptions of patient communications in student intern's clinical notes				
40		O	Articulates the patients' views during case consultations	Reports addressing patient views in student intern's case reviews				

Financial Implications Student interns will also demonstrate their *knowledge and application* of the financial implications of their clinical work by either discussing, describing, or incorporating concepts in their case consultations, planning notes, case presentations, consultation group discussions, and/or performance review meetings.

	Dimensions	Care behavioral anchors	Focus of evaluation	Proficient	Progressing	Missing	Not observed
41	F	Describes ways that work with patient populations optimizes practice financial resources	Reports addressing PHM approaches in student intern's case reviews				
42	F	Describes impact of behavioral involvement on shared financial responsibility with the medical team	Feedback from medical team that intern discusses appropriate use of financial resources in treatment planning				
43	F	Displays awareness of needed documentation for use of specific billing codes and appropriately completes documentation in notes	Review descriptions of billing codes in student intern's clinical notes				
44	F	Identifies how recommended treatments impact the utilization of resources	Reports addressing resource utilization in student intern's case reviews				

References

Burgess, A., McGregor, D., & Mellis, C. (2014). Applying established guidelines to team-based learning programs in medical schools: A systematic review. *Academic Medicine, 89*(4), 678–688.

Havyer, R., Wingo, M., Cornfere, N., Nelson, D., Halvoren, A., McDonald, F., et al. (2013). Teamwork assessment in internal medicine: A systematic review of validity evidence and outcomes. *Journal of General Internal Medicine, 29*(6), 894–910.

Hoge, M., Huey, L., & O'Connell, M. (2004). Best practices in behavioral health workforce education and training. *Administration and Policy in Mental Health, 32*(2), 91–106.

Hoge, M., Tondora, J., & Marrell, A. (2005). The fundamentals of workforce competency: Implications for behavioral health. *Administration and Policy in Mental Health, 32*(5/6), 509–531.

Hunter, C., & Goodie, J. (2010). Operational and clinical components for integrated-collaborative behavioral healthcare in the patient-centered medical home. *Families, Systems & Health, 28*(4), 306–321.

Hunter, C. L., Goodie, J. L., Oordt, M. S., & Dobmeyer, A. C. (2009). *Integrated behavioral health in primary care: Step-by-step guidance for assessment and intervention*. Washington, DC: American Psychological Association.

Institute of Medicine. (2015). *Measuring the impact of interprofessional education on collaborative practice and patient outcomes*. Retrieved from Washington, DC.

Interprofessional Education Collaborative Expert Panel. (2011). *Core competencies for interprofessional collaborative practice: Report of an expert panel*. Retrieved from Washington, DC: http://www.aacn.nche.edu/education-resources/IPECReport.pdf

Josiah Macy Jr. Foundation, & Interprofessional Education Collaborative. (2011). *Team-based competencies: Building a shared foundation for education and clinical practice*. Washington, DC: Interprofessional Education Collaborative.

Kinman, C., Gilchrist, E., Payne-Murphy, J., & Miller, B. (2015). *Provider- and practice-level competencies for integrated behavioral health in primary care: A literature review* (14–0073-EF). Retrieved from Rockville, MD: https://integrationacademy.ahrq.gov/sites/default/files/AHRQ_AcadLitReview.pdf

Merriam, S., & Bierema, L. (2014). *Adult learning: Linking theory and practice*. San Francisco: John Wiley.

Mitchell, P., Wynia, M., Golden, R., McNellis, B., Okun, S., Webb, C., et al. (2012). *Core principles & values of effective team-based health care*. Retrieved from Washington, DC: http://www.iom.edu/tbc

Peek, C. J. (2008). Planning care in the clinical, financial, and operational worlds. In R. Kessler & D. Stafford (Eds.), *Collaborative medicine case studies: Evidence in practice* (pp. 25–38). New York: Springer Science.

Robinson, P., & Reiter, J. (2016). *Behavioral consultation and primary care: A guide to integrating services* (2nd ed.). New York: Springer.

Rosenman, E., Ilgen, J., Shandro, J., Harper, A., & Fernandez, R. (2015). A systematic review of tools used to assess team leadership in health care action teams. *Academic Medicine, 90*(10), 1408–1422.

Stanhope, V., Solomon, P., Pernell-Arnold, A., Sands, R., & Bourjolly, J. (2005). Evaluating cultural competence among behavioral health professionals. *Psychiatric Rehabilitation Journal, 28*(3), 225–233.

Vygotsky, L. (1978). *Mind in society: The development of higher psychological processes*. Cambridge, MA: Harvard University Press.

Section III
Training the Workforce for Integrated BH Care

Chapter 4
PHM-Focused Healthcare Delivery

Sue Dahl-Popolizio and Stephanie Brennhofer

Chapter overview	
Domains	Population identification Patient identification through health assessments Risk stratification Engagement strategies Patient-centered interventions (group and/or individual) Program impact assessment/process improvement
Key points	Stakeholders must be considered in direction of education (e.g. patient, providers, employers, insurance companies, community members) Key components reflect goals of PHM: Increase access to care, maximize provider productivity, standardize procedures, prevention strategies, reduce the risk of exacerbation of conditions, improve overall health of the population, chronic care management, use of interprofessional teams for optimal workflow, and reduce overall costs
Foundational knowledge and skills	Ability to recognize and define populations and relevant stakeholders who will benefit from PHM programs, understand the current financial situation in healthcare requiring PHM programs, and recognize the benefit of the interprofessional primary care team
Student learning objectives (SLOs)	Upon completion of this chapter, the student will be able to: • Explain the evolution and purpose of PHM in the healthcare system • Describe the domains required for a successful PHM program and what they comprise • Describe the information required to determine workflows for a PHM program • Explain the evolution and purpose of PHM in integrated primary care • Explain the overarching goals of PHM programs • Explain training objectives as they relate to key concepts in PHM and relevant stakeholders • Explain how to create an effective PHM program • Identify key organizational support for developing PHM programs

S. Dahl-Popolizio (✉) · S. Brennhofer
Integrated Behavioral Health Programs, College of Health Solutions, Arizona State University, Phoenix, AZ, USA
e-mail: Sue.dahlpopolizio@asu.edu; Stephanie.Brennhofer@asu.edu

C. R. Macchi, R. Kessler (eds.), *Training to Deliver Integrated Care*,
https://doi.org/10.1007/978-3-319-78850-0_4

Chapter overview	
Instructional strategies	Provide didactics, case examples, and sample data sets to guide learner through the steps of developing, implementing, and evaluating a PHM program Assist learners with identifying and obtaining organizational-level support for accessing and reporting EHR data
Evaluating learning	Identify the key components of a PHM program Describe the steps of developing a PHM program Develop relationships with organizational leadership and QI specialists to design, implement, and evaluate a PHM program Obtain IT technical support for engaging with EHR data

Background

This chapter provides teaching strategies to educators who provide instruction regarding population health management (PHM) in an integrated primary care (IPC) setting. While many health assessment and treatment approaches target individual patients, a PHM approach is a broader view used to identify patient population needs, develop programs and services, and evaluate patient population health improvements. Addressing the health of a population meets the three dimensions of the Triple Aim: (1) improving the patient experience with healthcare, (2) improving the health of the overall population, and (3) reducing the per capita cost of healthcare. This chapter will primarily focus on effective PHM-related teaching strategies and resources needed to equip practitioners to address the second dimension of the Triple Aim.

History of Population Health Management Training Programs

Prior to the mid-twentieth century, health was measured primarily by disease prevalence and mortality rates. Similarly, PHM was reactionary-focused where the patient passively received care and the provider determined how disease was spread. In the mid-twentieth century, PHM was more of a reactionary response to acute disease. Providers were shifting toward treating and preventing the spread of disease, while beginning to educate the community on disease prevention and treatment. Primary care was introduced in the late twentieth century and was a mix between reactionary and preventative PHM. The public was educated on how disease spreads and given community control options (e.g., sanitation, hygiene, and immunizations). By the early twenty-first century, there was a shift toward proactive preventative care where providers identified high-risk patients before diseases set in and engaged patients in their healthcare to address their health behaviors. See Table 4.1 for more information on historical shifts over time.

Table 4.1 Historical shifts in population health management education

Phase 1 (precedes WWII)	Phase 2 (mid 20th century)	Phase 3 (late 20th century)	Phase 4 (early 21st century)
Reactionary			Preventative
Educate provider on how disease spreads	Educate provider on how to treat and prevent spread of disease, rather than disease occurrence	Educate community and patient on how disease is spread	Educate provider to identify at-risk individuals based on behavioral choices (e.g., smoking, diet) before medical issues arise
Patient is passive recipient of care	Being to educate community on how disease is spread	First public service campaigns/announcements regarding health (e.g., smoking, polio)	Provider stratifies patients based on risk level for appropriate prevention and/or intervention
	Identified populations at risk (not patients) for prevention and treatment, but role of provider is shared with community	Activate patient role in care – patient takes on more responsibility	

Key Conceptual and Operational Shifts in PHM

As the healthcare system has evolved, the shift from reactive to preventative healthcare has resulted in an increased need for developing, implementing, and evaluating effective PHM strategies. This increased demand for PHM programs has led to the need for training programs designed to equip providers with the skills to develop these strategies while including patients and their communities in the educational process. This shift intends to optimize the health of populations while minimizing the costs to the healthcare system.

Dimensions of Population Health Management

While there is no true consensus on defining population health, PHM, and public health, it is important to understand how PHM ties into both population and public health and how the determinants of health (e.g., behaviors/lifestyle, genetics, and community) influence all three (see Fig. 4.1). Population health is defined as "the health outcomes of a group of individuals, including the distribution of such outcomes within the group" (Kindig & Stoddart, 2003, p. 380). There are four pillars of population health: (1) quality and safety, (2) chronic condition management, (3) healthcare delivery, and (4) public health (Nash, Fabius, Skoufalos, Clarke, & Horowitz, 2016). PHM comprises pillars two through four and focuses on providing high-quality care for populations through collaborations of interdisciplinary teams; interventions to provide care can be population-based or one-on-one care. Public health is a component of population health, which focuses on the health of an entire population through healthcare quality and access, but is not

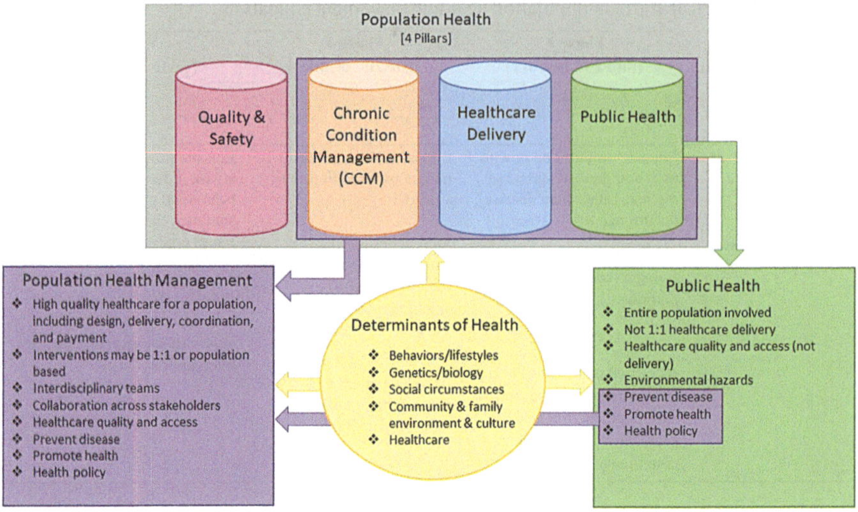

Fig. 4.1 Relationships among population health, PHM, and public health

healthcare delivery. Public health encompasses interactions between behavior and health within the context of the social determinants of health and environmental influences on health. These factors have an influence on the distribution and the interventions and policies that affect these determinants (Nash et al., 2016).

Key components of PHM in IPC include increasing access to care, maximizing provider productivity, standardizing procedures, engaging in prevention strategies, reducing the risk of exacerbation of conditions, improving overall health of the population, using interprofessional teams for optimal workflow, and reducing overall costs. Considering the collaborative, team-based approach of IPC, the concept of PHM fits well into this setting. The overall goal of any PHM program design in IPC is dependent upon the stakeholders involved, including patients, care providers, employers, insurance companies, communities, and the administrators of various types of healthcare organizations. Effective programs are tailored to meet the specific needs of a population in a cost-effective manner. Although the desired overall outcome of improving the health of the population is clear, the method of achieving this outcome is not specifically defined. Population health approaches vary based upon the mission and goals of the stakeholders and the perspective of the specific program or organization implementing a PHM strategy. These programs may focus on the use of technology to manage the health of a population, community resources and programs, or patient programs within IPC practices. The remaining sections of this chapter address methods to train IPC teams on each key PHM component that is employed within IPC settings.

Factors to Consider for Effective PHM Programs, Core Competencies, and Training

In IPC, the process of creating a PHM program must include strategies to address the integrated healthcare PHM domains, which are well outlined by Population Health Alliance (PHA), formerly the Care Continuum Alliance (CCA). First, identify the target population and specific patients within the population. Next, stratify patients based on risk and place them in the appropriate level of care. Then, engage the population in the program, provide interventions consistent with risk level, and assess outcomes and effectiveness of the program (CCA, 2012).

Collaboration among the multiple professionals on the primary care team is critical to efficiently and cost-effectively meet the needs of the population in IPC. A team-based approach to implementing a successful PHM program requires the provision of training that defines and clarifies the complimentary roles of each team member. The key components of a comprehensive IPC PHM program target specific goals. PHM training program design, implementation, and evaluation is based upon aligning those goals with targeted stakeholder interests and training objectives that address provider competencies and skills development. The training program begins by assisting the learner with identifying the problem that the PHM program is intended to address and the stakeholders who should be involved in identifying the goals of that program. Next, the training program guides the process of conducting an assessment of available resources and determines the best PHM strategy that is suited to the organization or target population. An emphasis is placed on effective ways to engage stakeholders to secure stakeholder buy-in at this early stage. Success of PHM programs relies heavily on the stakeholders' belief that the program benefits clearly outweigh the program costs.

Training Strategies to Address Practitioner Performance Barriers to Integration

Training strategies must address the barriers associated with implementing PHM programs. One such barrier is reflected in providers' and administrators' difficulty in making the shift from individual care to population-based care. This shift involves cognitively transitioning from a reactive approach to individual healthcare to a risk management and prevention approach that focuses on improving the health of the population. It is critical to teach providers how to use data to support their claims. They can use information from the literature, from similar practices, or from their own practice. Electronic health records (EHRs) are ideal sources of data in a clinical practice setting.

The first step to educating providers on how to make these shifts in thinking is to determine the prevalence of a specific condition within a population. Common chronic illnesses can be effectively treated at the population level. The providers

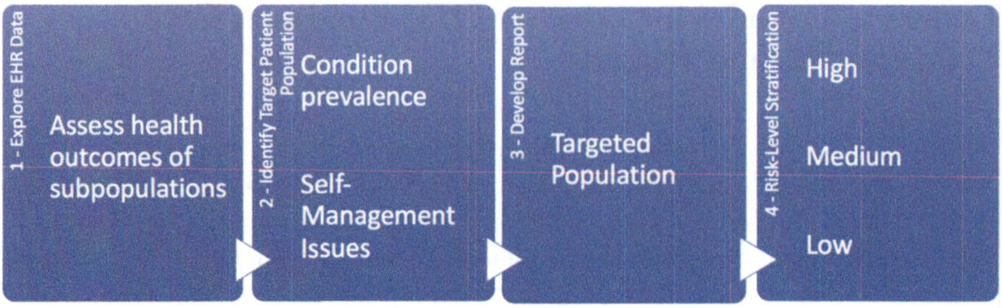

Fig. 4.2 PHM patient identification and stratification steps

must first learn to target common chronic diseases that are currently associated with poor patient self-management strategies. This targeted focus facilitates a natural shift to addressing the needs of that specific population. Next, teach the provider to stratify the population based on risk level identified through health assessments. As they grasp the concept of stratification, the next phase in PHM is to place patients in the level of care that corresponds with their identified risk level. This placement includes low risk and prevention as part of the overall PHM approach (Fig. 4.2).

Team membership and roles related to PHM have not yet been clarified, making full implementation of interprofessional team-based care difficult. Instruct providers to educate themselves about the roles, training, and scope of practice of the different professions they may find on an interprofessional team. Chapter 3 discusses several professions and their function on the primary care team. Providers can research, interact, and engage with the different professions they find on their team or are interested in including on their team. This interaction will foster more efficient and effective use of team members. The leader of a PHM program should understand the potential contributions of each team member so that each member is able to work at their highest skill level to maximize productivity and provider satisfaction, while meeting patient and team needs.

Obtaining reimbursement frequently poses a barrier to PHM implementation. Reimbursement strategies for PHM vary depending on the reimbursement structure of the organization. Different reimbursement models include fee for service, bundled payments, quality incentive payment system, capitation, and more. Reimbursement for PHM programs, including preventative programs, in the residual fee-for-service models is challenging and can be a deterrent to utilizing PHM programs that depend on nonreimbursable professionals. Since prevention and identification of at-risk patients or those who are not yet sick is at the core of PHM, reimbursement for PHM programs is difficult to obtain in a traditional, reactionary intervention environment. It is important to educate regarding which professions are able to obtain reimbursement for services in the region where they will be working, as this can vary among states and regions. The providers and administrators must learn how to use common procedural terminology (CPT) codes when appropriate. The different billable professionals should know how to bill for the services they provide. Providers and administrators should meet with these professionals to determine the most effective and cost-effective use of the billable professionals' skills in the primary care setting. If the practice uses non-billable entities, they must be able to explain why they are doing so and how their use of these non-billable entities is cost-effective. It is possible that the cost of some non-billable entities is considered an overhead expense in the budget. In this case, the non-billable entity can track the measures (e.g., interventions provided, population served, decrease in number of office or emergency room visits, or decrease in prescriptions required) which demonstrate their productivity and program effectiveness.

The teaching approach depends on the stakeholder. Ideally the educator will be aware of the resources and culture of the community in which the providers they are training will practice and gear their training toward the stakeholders in that community. If the educator is providing general education, they will provide general information on the issues discussed above. PHM programs, when used to address the needs of the whole person in the primary care setting, include the provision of behavioral health services. Many practices do not have staff or systems in place to address this aspect of patient need. They can determine which professional is best suited to provide this integrated behavioral health service based on professional background, billing needs of the practice, patient needs of the practice, and level of education around the provision of behavioral healthcare in a primary care setting of the professional they are interested in employing for this purpose.

Training or Skill Acquisition Needed to Effectively Implement PHM

Practitioner Performance of Core Competency Skills The provision of PHM programs is becoming a core competency for all healthcare providers. Although a set of core competencies for organizations and providers providing PHM programs specifically has not been established, we can begin with the core competencies proposed for IPC practices (see Table 2 in Chap. 3) that readily apply to those providing PHM in the primary care setting as well. However, there are competencies specific to the provision of PHM in primary care that are not included in any of these core competency lists. Educators must ensure that the providers and administrators who they are training to function in integrated behavioral health settings obtain competency in these areas.

Team-Based Care Approach to PHM Traditionally, providers have functioned in silos, working side by side in many cases, but unaware of what the other providers were doing and the overlapping areas in their respective scopes of practice. For optimal effectiveness of PHM, all providers and staff should be educated regarding the full scopes of practice of their colleagues. This training should reflect the *top of the license* model where all team members use their unique skills and do not engage in low-skilled intake screenings and measurements (e.g., obtaining weight, height, and blood pressure readings). When health professionals are using skills specific to their license (e.g., counseling patients to address behavioral health issues or care management tasks), physicians are able to work at the top of their licenses as well.

When the physician's time is used judiciously, the physician is available to attend to more of the most seriously ill patients presenting to the clinic, a concept critical to the success of a PHM program. When everyone is working at the top of their license, the practice is as productive as possible, and the patients have as much access to the care they need as possible. When done well, this leads to increased health of the population, increased patient satisfaction with their level of care, and improved per capita costs as patients will return less frequently, and conditions will not exacerbate to the level where the patient returns or goes to a higher level of care such as the emergency room or urgent care. The actual PHM programs best suited for a practice vary among practice settings, regions, patients served, and payment structure. Table 4.2 provides a general template to plan the structure of PHM programs and develop the best workflow based on professionals present in the practice to meet presenting patient needs.

Performance Impact on Utilization, Costs, and Return on Investment (ROI) By implementing an effective PHM program, there will be an increase in utilization of some services, with the goal of decreasing utilization of other, more expensive services. This is especially true in an IPC setting when all interprofessional team members are working effectively at the top of their licenses. For instance, in the patient population with uncontrolled diabetes, the cost of providing behavioral health services, historically, would be seen as an additional cost to the practice. In an integrated setting, the patient sees the behavioral health provider instead of the physician, to address their healthcare needs related to their behaviors. The resulting cost of the behavioral health provider visit is less than the cost of the PCP visit and more effectively addresses the patient's behavioral issues. Also, patients receiving more effective, less expensive levels of care may be more likely to experience a reduction of symptom exacerbations and avoid the need for accessing more expensive services (e.g., hospitalizations, diagnostic testing, and referrals to specialists).

To determine the cost effectiveness of a program, training programs should equip learners with the skills needed to calculate the ROI of programs and services. In PHM, ROI can be determined by looking at financial gain or cost savings. It is critical that providers and administrators be educated regarding the difference between these two different concepts. Financial ROI is determined by examining the amount of program costs and comparing it to the revenue that the program generated. Cost savings is determined by identifying a reduction in utilization of medical services. In PHM, this is typically due to improved patient identification and engagement in PHM programs, which result in a reduction in expensive healthcare utilization due to improved self-management skills.

IPC operates under the premise that providing less expensive behavioral health services decreases the number of patient primary care visits. As patients develop increasingly effective self-management skills, those patients more effectively

Table 4.2 PHM development planning guide

Patient identification		
Patients can be identified by: • Primary care physician (PCP) diagnosis • EHR data • Any provider or staff noting patient needs or requests suggest a diagnosis appropriate for a PHM program (e.g., patient calls requesting referral for shoes due to diabetic neuropathy, automatic referral to diabetes PHM program)		
Referral to PHM program		
Health assessment • Use assessment appropriate for target diagnosis/population • Use providers in the practice with the skill set to administer the diagnosis • Use for risk stratification level and initial placement in appropriate level of care • Use post-intervention to: – Assess effectiveness of intervention – Assess patient progress and move to lower or higher level of care based on outcomes		
Low risk	**Moderate risk**	**High risk**
Provide: Education regarding: wellness/prevention strategies	Provide: Education regarding: • Necessary lifestyle changes • Medication adherence • Community supports Intervention: • Groups for education and coping strategies, lifestyle modification, and behavioral health issues. Group frequency and duration dependent on condition and risk level • Individual outreach as needed type, frequency, and duration dependent on condition and risk level	Provide: Education regarding: • Disease management • Necessary lifestyle changes • Medication adherence • Community supports Intervention: • Supplement intervention in moderate level of care with disease management • 1:1 intervention supplements group interventions • Frequent individual outreach to ensure optimal carry-over of instructions
Patient evaluation		
Re-assess: In 6 months–1 year typically	Re-assess more frequently: In 3 months or less	Re-assess at least monthly
Program evaluation		
Track patient outcomes to determine effectiveness of the program. Use outcomes to identify processes in the program to improve		

$$\text{ROI} = \frac{\text{Gain from program} - \text{Cost of program}}{\text{Cost of program}}$$

$$\text{ROI} = \frac{[\$70{,}427.50 \text{ (from BHP)} + \$73{,}530 \text{ (from PCP)}] - \$65{,}000 \text{ (BCP salary \& benefits)}}{\$65{,}000 \text{ (\$50k BCP salary \& 30\% benefits)}}$$

$$\text{ROI} = \frac{\$143{,}957.50 - \$65{,}000 = \$78{,}957.5}{\$65{,}000} = 1.21$$

ROI = 1.21 (for every $1 spent on the BHP, $1.21 additional is earned by the clinic)

Fig. 4.3 Financial ROI

$$\text{ROI} = \frac{\text{Cost savings attributed to program}}{\text{Cost of program}}$$

$$\text{ROI} = \frac{\$1{,}886{,}500 \text{ (reduction in unnecessary ER visits and PCP visits)}}{\$65{,}000 \text{ (\$50k BCP salary \& 30\% benefits)}} = 29$$

ROI = 29 (for every $1 spent on the BCP, $29 is saved in avoidance of healthcare costs due to overutilization of more expensive services)

Fig. 4.4 Cost-saving ROI

adhere to medical instructions. Practices using PHM programs can more effectively identify patients across the continuum of care severity and can efficiently and cost-effectively address the needs of the population. For example, since PCP visits are billed at a higher rate in a fee-for-service environment, other environments may initially suggest a loss of revenue. Consider again the *top of the license* principle. If the use of the behavioral health provider allows the PCP to see patients who truly require the skillset of the PCP, they will be billing for higher-level visits that are reimbursed at a higher rate. The increased revenue generated by the increased number of these higher-level visits helps offset the cost of the behavioral health services. Fee-for-service reimbursement depends on the professional providing the behavioral health service, available CPT codes dictated by license type, and third-party payer plans.

When training administrators, practice managers, and others involved in the billing process about ROI in an IPC setting, it is critical that education focuses on comparing financial and cost-saving ROIs. Below are two simple but effective formulas to educate on what to include and how to determine both financial ROI and cost-saving ROI. The example is simplified as well for illustrative purposes (Figs. 4.3 and 4.4).

Measurement of Effective PHM Training Approaches

Typically, outcomes of PHM are measured after long-term, one year or more, use of the program. It is critical to assess long-term outcomes to determine the overall effectiveness of the program. However, measuring the effectiveness of the program does not provide feedback regarding the effectiveness of the treatment offered by the providers. To assess training effectiveness, as well as the effectiveness of a PHM program, change in patient status and change in level of care can be used as metrics of program effectiveness. Arguably, significant changes in status and level of care will not be seen if the program creators have not been effectively trained. Using the health assessments appropriate for the condition before and after inclusion in the PHM program can provide information regarding the effectiveness of the intervention. To clearly measure effectiveness, set specific measurable goals with a time line; for example, there will be a 25% reduction in PCP visits among patients after participating in the program for 6 months. After a specified point in the program (e.g., 1 year after program initiation), assess whether goals have been met.

There are many ways to determine the effectiveness of training more specifically, and the method should reflect the student and educational setting. In a didactic course, create a grading rubric that evaluates learner performance related to specific instructional strategies addressing each step of a PHM program:

- Identifying and targeting a patient subpopulation
- Risk stratification
- Engagement strategies
- Patient-centered interventions

Learners must be instructed to develop relationships with key members within the organization (e.g. IT, care managers, clinical leadership, QI specialists) who have the expertise and can provide the support needed to access the available data in the EHR. In clinical settings, some possible data points that may be used to determine the effectiveness of a PHM program include:

- Number of patients referred to the PHM program
- Health assessment scores after participation in the program, or at set points in the ongoing program
- Number of emergency room visits in the target population after the intervention
- Change in number of office visits in the target population after the intervention

Case Example Template for PHM Training Program

The PHA provides a guide for PHM implementation and evaluation (CCA, 2012) and is an excellent resource for PHM developers. This section provides the essential components or domains to consider and/or include in an effective PHM program, consistent with recommendations of the CCA guide; they are presented in the recommended step-by-step order. When training providers, encourage them to consider the needs and culture of their target population, envisioning patients they have seen or case studies they have read. Instruct them to consider resources and personnel available, reimbursement structure, and financial requirements of the practice. Although the healthcare system is moving away from fee for service, this reimbursement model is still the most common reimbursement model in healthcare, so whether reimbursement is required for PHM program sustainability is an important factor to consider when developing the program. All of these considerations will help the program developer create the workflow pattern that fits best into the practice.

Population Identification Clearly describe the target population, which can be defined by diagnosis, geographic area, members of a practice, or subscribers to an insurance plan. Once the population is defined, patients can be identified with regular patient health screenings, automatic physician referral based on diagnosis, diagnoses obtained from an EHR, and more. The use of EHR is recommended whenever possible. This is done by using health assessments that are evidence-based, and their use is conducive to the fast pace of the primary care clinic. Some examples include: Patient Health Questionnaire 2 or 9 (PHQ-2 or PHQ-9) for depression, the Duke (general health profile), and Morisky Medication Adherence Scale (MMAS). Choose the assessments based on the target illness or population for your PHM program.

Risk Stratification Risk stratification is most commonly determined by using established health assessment thresholds to determine the most appropriate level of care for the patient. For instance, these are the score thresholds identified by the developers of the assessment PHQ-9:

- Level 1 (low risk) = minimal depression (5–9 score)
- Level 2 (moderate risk) = moderate depression (10–14 score)
- Level 3 (severe risk) = moderately severe to severe depression (≥15 score)

Risk stratification can include comorbid conditions as well. For example:

- Level 1 (low risk) = minimal depression (5–9 score) and prediabetes based on HbA1c (5.7–6.4%)
- Level 2 (moderate risk) = moderate depression (10–14 score) and controlled diabetes based on HbA1c (6.5–7.9%)
- Level 3 (severe risk) = moderately severe to severe depression (≥15 score) and uncontrolled diabetes diagnosis based on HbA1c (8.0% or higher)

It is imperative the system identifies all patients who can benefit from the PHM program and places them in the most appropriate level of care. The higher outcome measure will dictate the level of care the patient is classified in. For example, a patient presenting with moderate risk for depression (Level 2) and prediabetes (Level 1) would be a Level 2 classification because one of the comorbid conditions ranked as a Level 2. Likewise, a patient with low risk for depression (Level 1) and controlled diabetes (Level 2) would also be a Level 2 classification.

Engagement Strategies It is critical to determine which outreach strategy will facilitate enrollment and participation of the target population. Without effective patient engagement in the program, even the best program will be ineffective. Providers and administrators who create PHM programs must be trained to evaluate the potential participants. Social determinants of health including culture, social groups, superstitions, beliefs and factors that contribute to personal motivation must be considered when developing a PHM program to ensure patient engagement.

Another critical factor for patient engagement is marketing and outreach. There are many basic strategies that increase program awareness. For instance, educate the office staff to refer appropriate patients to the program and teach them how to add information regarding the program to the practice website. Additionally, peer partners or the buddy system can be an effective engagement strategy. Effective engagement strategies lead to an increased sense of the provider's interest in the patient's health, resulting in improved patient experience. Outreach to all levels of the identified population reduces symptom exacerbations, which decreases the cost of care while addressing the healthcare needs of the population. Again, the Triple Aim is addressed.

Patient-Centered Interventions Use risk stratification levels to place patients into corresponding levels of care in a timely manner. These levels of care reflect the treatment intervention a provider will offer to patients in the different risk stratification levels. Care can be provided in one-on-one or group settings, depending on the type and severity of the condition addressed. Treatment can range from basic educational or preventative health actions to direct patient care for more severely ill patients. All levels should facilitate improved self-management skills. The level of risk dictates the amount, type, and frequency of intervention. Possible interventions appropriate for PHM programs include overall case management, behavioral modification strategies to improve medication compliance, group and brief individual counseling, physical activity groups or strategies, and strategies to improve diet for patients with chronic diseases. There will be more patients in the lower levels of care; these patients will need less hands-on intervention and less frequent interaction. The fewer patients in the higher levels of care will need more hands-on care and direct intervention. Plan an intervention for each level of care identified.

Program Impact Assessment/Process Improvement Intervention Goals Providers and administrators must be trained to create realistic, attainable, and measurable intervention goals for each level of care that represent overarching program goals. All goals must be identifiable, objective, and measurable. Use the acronym SMART to ensure goals are appropriate (S: specific, M: measurable, A: achievable, R: realistic/relevant, T: time based). For instance, a program goal could be that 75% of patients in Level 3 will be de-escalated to Level 2 within 3 months of starting the intervention. There must be subsequent patient goals to be able to achieve this program goal. Perhaps a patient goal could be that a patient in Level 3 will participate in 2 weekly groups per month for 3 months. While these are generic examples, they are clearly objective and measurable.

With any PHM program, there should be general expected outcomes of the program stated in terms of change in pre- and post-intervention measure. Anticipated outcomes are based on findings in the literature regarding how patients in the target population respond to the intervention. Assist PHM developers to focus on creating a reasonable program based on evidence found in the literature and organizational and government websites. An effective process improvement strategy begins by reviewing goals that are partially met or anticipated outcomes that do not reflect the expected changes. The results of these reviews are used to modify the interventions.

The information and resources presented in this chapter provide the educator with teaching strategies to facilitate understanding and development of PHM programs in IPC. The PHM approach in IPC will help healthcare providers focus on the second dimension of the triple aim. However, as explained in this chapter, when used effectively, PHM in IPC can advance the movement toward achieving all three goals of the Triple Aim by (1) improving the patient experience with healthcare, (2) improving the health of the overall population, and (3) reducing the per capita cost of healthcare.

References

Care Continuum Alliance. (2012). *Implementation and evaluation: A population health guide for primary care models*. Retrieved from http://www.populationhealthalliance.org

Kindig, D., & Stoddart, G. (2003). What is population health? *American Journal of Public Health, 93*(3), 380–383.

Nash, D. B., Fabius, R. J., Skoufalos, A., Clarke, J. L., & Horowitz, M. R. (2016). *Population health: Creating a culture of wellness*. Burlington, MA: Jones & Bartlett.

Chapter 5
Quality Improvement, Performance Management, and Outcomes: Lean Six Sigma for Integrated Behavioral Health

Ronald O'Donnell and Rodger Kessler

Chapter overview	
Domains	*Competencies design and implementation of Lean Six Sigma quality improvement strategies and techniques*
Key points	*The core competencies for quality improvement and performance management in integrated behavioral healthcare require approaches consistent with new models of value-based care and reimbursement. Quality improvement strategies and techniques based on Lean Six Sigma are well-suited to meet this need*
Foundational knowledge and skills	*Ability to design, deliver, and evaluate a Lean Six Sigma quality improvement program in integrated behavioral healthcare settings*
Student learning objectives (SLOs)	*Complete a value stream map and analysis* *Complete a plan-do-study-act cycle* *Construct a control chart* *Create an A3 report* *Complete a rapid improvement event*
Instructional strategies	*Lecture, discussion, digital video media, assigned readings, role-play, and presentations*
Evaluating learning	*Quizzes, written assignments, grading discussions, and presentations*

R. O'Donnell (✉) · R. Kessler
Integrated Behavioral Health Programs, College of Health Solutions, Arizona State University, Phoenix, AZ, USA
e-mail: Ronald.ODonnell@asu.edu; Rodger.kessler@asu.edu

C. R. Macchi, R. Kessler (eds.), *Training to Deliver Integrated Care*,
https://doi.org/10.1007/978-3-319-78850-0_5

Introduction

A key characteristic of healthcare reform is an increased focus on improving provider quality of care, accountability for quality via performance measurement, and aligning provider reimbursement to meet national and regional quality of care performance targets. These healthcare goals reflected the call to achieve the "Triple Aim" of improved patient experience of care, improved population health, and reduced cost of care (Berwick, Nolan, & Whittington, 2008). Berwick et al. (2008) noted that in spite of spending on healthcare that is nearly double that of the next most costly nation, the United States is ranked very low globally on many health indicators, such as life expectancy and infant mortality (Institute of Medicine, 2001).

One reason for poor quality is the gap between the care that is actually provided and evidence-based standards (Blumenthal & McGinnis, 2015). There is significant variability among healthcare providers in the degree of fidelity to the evidence base for practice, and the existing business case for healthcare delivery is misaligned, with a focus on payment for volume in the fee-for-service model of reimbursement without attention to the quality of care, outcomes, or costs (Bao et al., 2017). The need to balance quality and cost has led to the emergence of value-based payment (VBP) models of provider reimbursement designed to pay providers based on predetermined quality and efficiency targets (Bao et al., 2017).

This chapter is designed to prepare primary care integrated behavioral health provider (BHP) clinicians and managers to practice Lean Six Sigma quality improvement strategies and techniques. The BHP is faced with the challenge of introducing the primary care behavioral health model (Robinson & Reiter, 2016) into a primary care system that is pressured with many changes in practice management associated with the Triple Aim. This includes the transition to VBP models and adapting the patient-centered medical home (PCMH) model. These pressures leave the primary care workforce reporting widespread burnout and dissatisfaction, leading for a call to add improving the work life of healthcare providers as a fourth, or "quadruple aim," to the Triple Aim of healthcare (Bodenheimer & Sinsky, 2014).

In addition to these challenges, the BHP must also address the need to develop, implement, and evaluate effective models of primary care behavioral health. A recent survey by the National Committee for Quality Assurance found that less than 40% of certified patient-centered medical homes have any mental health or behavioral care (Kessler et al., 2014). When BHPs are added to primary care, they are often not integrated into the practice workflow (Kessler et al., 2014). The field lacks the knowledge and competencies about how to implement integrated behavioral healthcare into primary care (Kessler, 2012). A recent study noted a lack of a unified model of how to manage scheduling and productivity for primary care-based BHPs (Thomas-Henkel, Hamblin, & Hendricks, 2015). In sum, the BHP is faced with the challenge of implementing integrated behavioral health programs into primary care clinics that are struggling to improve quality and efficiency, lack expertise in developing workflows to support integration, and providers who are stressed and dissatisfied.

Lean Six Sigma strategies and techniques for improvement seem ideally suited to prepare BHPs to effectively improve quality, outcomes, and reduce provider stress. Lean Six Sigma approaches were developed in the manufacturing sector to improve the efficiency of production processes and have been widely applied in healthcare (Deblois & Lepanto, 2016). Lean is based on the Toyota Production System to eliminate waste from the production process (Womack & Jones, 2003). Womack and Jones (2003) describes five fundamental components of Lean: specify a value, identify the value stream, crate the value stream map of flow in the process, let customers pull from the process, and seek perfection. Six Sigma was developed by Motorola, with an emphasis on quality control tools such as statistical methods to reduce error and minimize variability in processes and outcomes (Joint Commission on the Accreditation of Healthcare Organizations, 2008). Lean and Six Sigma are combined into a single approach referred to as Lean Six Sigma (Glasgow, Scott-Caziewell, & Kaboli, 2010). The goal of Lean Six Sigma is to improve quality and outcomes of care by decreasing waste and improving efficiency and by developing standard processes and workflows that support evidence-based practice. As a bonus, Lean Six Sigma relies upon engagement of frontline staff in the improvement process, enabling those with the clearest view of workflow problems to contribute to effective improvements. This empowerment can help reduce stress and burnout as providers unite in a team-based approach to improve the quality, efficiency, and their satisfaction with primary care processes. In effect, Lean Six Sigma strategies and techniques support team-based care critical to the PCMH model, improved outcomes and efficiencies required by VBP, and opportunities to improve workforce burnout – in effect, to achieve the quadruple aim.

Lean Six Sigma is conducted by a primary care team representing different work functions led by an expert in applying the strategies and techniques. The process includes activities such as creating a diagram of current processes and outcomes, identifying sources of waste and inefficiency, and conducting a root cause analysis to identify problems. The team then identifies potential solutions and plans to implement a system redesign project. Lean Six Sigma emphasizes system redesign projects that have clearly defined activities, objective measures of processes and outcomes, and adaptation to the local culture of the healthcare system. Lean Six Sigma relies on data visualization tools to evaluate and monitor performance, such as workflow diagrams, diagrams to illustrate problems, graphs and figures to track outcomes, and a summary sheet of the action plan and results. These visual tools are designed to facilitate shared understanding among the team members and to aid in visual tracking of targeted outcomes (Delisle, 2016).

The purpose of this chapter is to prepare the BHP learner to master key competencies in Lean Six Sigma. The breadth and depth of Lean Six Sigma training and education approaches are beyond the scope of this chapter. For example, lengthy certification for Lean Six Sigma requires extensive periods of study and practice. This chapter will present a sample of key competencies in Lean Six Sigma that will enable the BHP learner to successfully implement improvement efforts.

Integrated Behavioral Health Lean Six Sigma Competencies

Lean is based on five principles (Delisle, 2015). *Define value* is the first principle. This includes a well-defined scope of the project that includes a detailed description and project boundaries. A flowchart or process map called the SIPOC is completed that identifies the *supplier*; the person or department that initiates the process; the *inputs* that are the materials, resources, or information required to execute the process; the *process* steps to convert inputs to outputs; the *output*, a product, service, or outcome resulting from the process; and the *customer* that receives the outcome (SIPOC) (Delisle, 2015).

Value is defined through the customer's eyes, based on receiving the right care that the customer wants, when they want it, and in the right amount (Chalice, 2007). In integrated behavioral health, the customer is typically the PCP and/or the patient. There are three categories of value in a SIPOC: value-added (VA), non-value-added (NVA), or non-value-added but required (NVA-R) by an agency or other entity (Delisle, 2015). A VA activity is defined as something the customer is willing to pay for, effectively changes the product or service being delivered, and is completed correctly the first time without error (Delisle, 2015). A NVA is synonymous with waste in healthcare. A NOA-R activity does not add value, but it is required by an outside agency, such as an accreditation body in healthcare. The goal of Lean is to reduce waste and improve efficiency in healthcare. Lean identifies eight types of waste using the acronym DOWNTIME (Delisle, 2015):

Defects:	Activity caused by rework, errors, and incorrect information
Overproduction:	Production that is in excess, too soon, or faster than the process requires
Waiting:	Time wasted waiting for the next step in the process
Non-utilized talent:	Underutilizing the skills or intellect of employees engaged in the process
Transportation:	Unnecessary movement of items in the process
Inventory:	Excess products or items that are not utilized in the process
Motion:	Unnecessary movement by the employee in the process
Extra processing:	Any extraneous activity that is not required in the process

Map the value stream is the second principle of Lean (Delisle, 2015). The first step is to create a SIPOC of the current state, i.e., what the process is like as it actually happens now. The value stream map is completed by actually walking through, observing, and recording the process. Data is entered on the duration of each step in the process, waiting time (waste) between steps, and the percentage of time that each step is completed correctly. The data collected is then recorded on an updated process map called the value stream map (VSM). The value stream map uses symbols to identify VA, NVA, and NVA-R and includes a number of calculations designed to quantify these activities (Fig. 5.1).

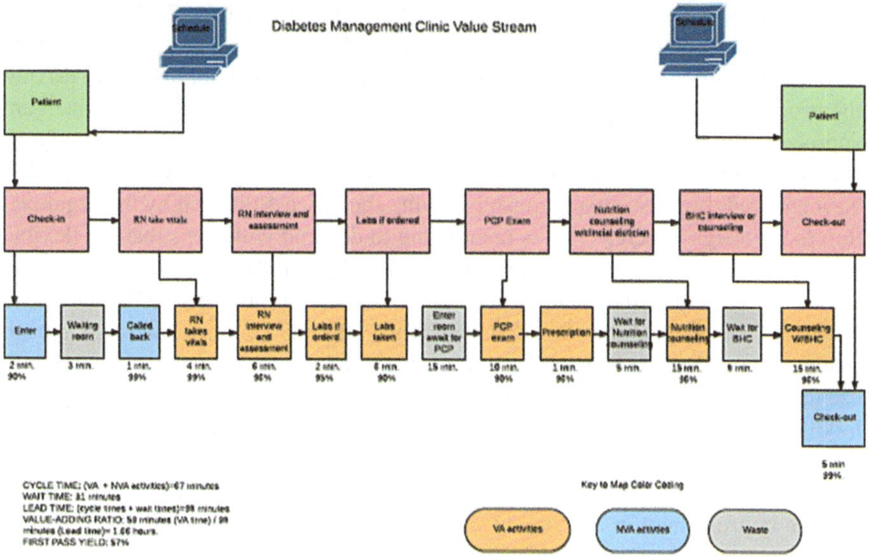

Fig. 5.1 Value stream map for diabetes clinic patient visit (From: Napier, 2017)

The next step is for the team to analyze the VSM using a process value analysis. This analysis is used to analyze ideas to improve efficiency by reducing waste such as waiting time.

Establish flow is the third principle of Lean and is comprised of three elements: determine customer demand, balance the process, and standardize the work (Delisle, 2015). Flow, a critical component of Lean strategy, is based on doing things correctly the first time while reducing waste in the process. In continuous flow, providers, patients, information, and equipment move along the process with accuracy and minimal waste, resulting in more VA than NVA activities. Determining customer demand is a critical step and requires the BHP to project how many patients will be seen on an average day. The takt time calculation is used to determine customer demand. It is calculated based on the daily available time (BHP hours/minutes in the clinic) divided by the number of patients, adjusting for breaks and lunch. Next, to balance the process, the BHP will analyze the amount of time it takes to complete each step with a process value analysis. The process value analysis is used to evaluate how to improve each step by increasing VA and decreasing NVA. The last component is to standardize the work, meaning to create consistent processes that reduce variability (Delisle, 2015). Creating standards is necessary to document the best way to complete a process. Standards are necessary to ensure that all staff are following best practices and serve as a basis to determine how to improve processes. The steps in creating standards include identifying problems or sources of variation, documenting and evaluating the current state to find ways to improve efficiency and reduce waste, training staff in the standards, implementation, and monitoring, and evaluating over time for continuous improvement (Delisle, 2015).

Implement pull is the fourth principle of Lean (Delisle, 2015). Push and pull are manufacturing concepts to describe the transition from one step in the process to the next. Push refers to the input (e.g., physician referral, patient appointment) driving the process without regard to the resources available. Pull refers to a downstream approach in which resources are prepared in anticipation of the demand so that as the patient transitions from one step to the other chances of delay, waiting, or other waste are reduced. Essentially, push is having the process dictated by the organization fixed design, whereas pull is responding to demand with steps that are flexible in order to meet changes in demand, such as a higher number of patient visits to the BHP on a particular day than on average. For example, if the BHP scheduled 6 1-h-fixed patient appointments per day and the PCPs had 12 warm hands-off, a push system would result in patient waits or rescheduling. In a pull system, the BHP will use flexible appointment scheduling to keep some appointments open each day, may modify the goals of a session with an individual patient when there are many patients waiting to be seen, or may use a group check-in to manage multiple patients at once.

Strive for perfection is the fifth principle of Lean, referring to the focus on continuous improvement in and organization (Delisle, 2015). There are three components to strive for perfection: identify root causes, error-proof processes, and sustain improvements. The Lean approach is designed to analyze problems by carefully observing and analyzing processes in order to identify and understand underlying root causes (Delisle, 2015). The root cause is the issue underlying problems in processes such as rework or waste. The root cause is identified with the gemba walk in the work area, interviewing staff and observing providers and patients. Once the root cause of an error is identified, the issues are isolated in order to develop a successful improvement strategy.

There are techniques designed to help identify root causes. The five why's are designed to explore root causes by probing below the presenting symptom. The symptom or problem is identified, and the question "why" is repeated five times, each time diving deeper into the process step details in order to identify the root cause. A fishbone diagram, also called Ishikawa or cause-and-effect diagram, guides systematic evaluation of the problem under analysis. This technique lends itself to brainstorming activities in a group/team. The steps to building a fishbone diagram include selecting the problem, creating the body (structure), labeling the categories (e.g., human resources, measurement, methods, equipment), and brainstorming potential causes (Delisle, 2015) (Fig. 5.2).

Error-proofing is intended to identify and evaluate errors as a learning opportunity and a chance design the error out of the process (Delisle, 2015). Quality checks are built into the process to prevent errors so that each step is completed correctly the first time and every time (Delisle, 2015). Human error is a common source of problems in healthcare processes. Common reasons for errors include lack of training or experience, forgetfulness, lack of standards, intentional errors, or inadvertent errors. Sustaining improvements requires a system of monitoring and reevaluating processes in order to make corrections as needed.

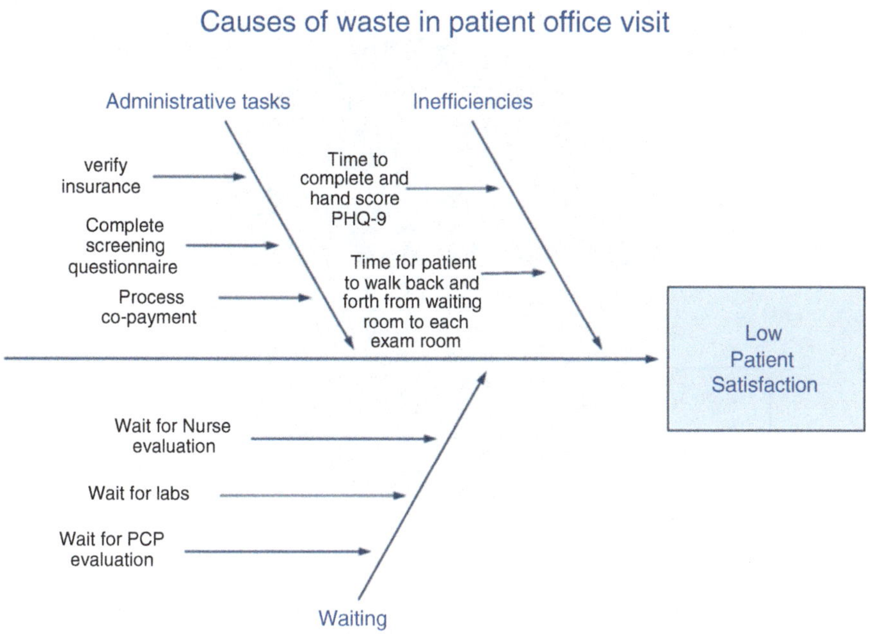

Fig. 5.2 Causes of waste in a patient office visit

Managing Lean Six Sigma improvement projects is often conducted using the IHI Performance Improvement Model (Ogrinc et al., 2012). There are three key questions in the model for improvement:

- What are we trying to accomplish (the aim)?
- How will we know a change is an improvement (the measures)?
- What changes can we make that will result in an improvement?

Once these questions are answered, the plan-do-study-act (PDSA) cycle is used to design improvement activities and test them. The PDSA cycle is shorthand for designing a plan to test the change (plan), implementing the test (do), observing and evaluating the results (study), and deciding what changes should be made to improve the process (act) (Fig. 5.3).

Control charts are commonly used approach to monitoring and evaluating performance metrics over time and predict what will happen in the future (IHI). Traditional pre- and post-intervention comparisons of performance metrics provide weak demonstration of changes over time (IHI). Control charts use the concept of replication, the process of evaluating successive results, to evaluate the pattern of changes over time to test the intervention. They use replication for analysis to show whether or not an intervention produces a pattern of change in the observed results (IHI). A control chart is comprised of a center line on a graph that is the mean score of the change measure, with lines above and below called upper control limit (UCL) and lower control limit (LCL). The UCL and LCL represent boundaries that are

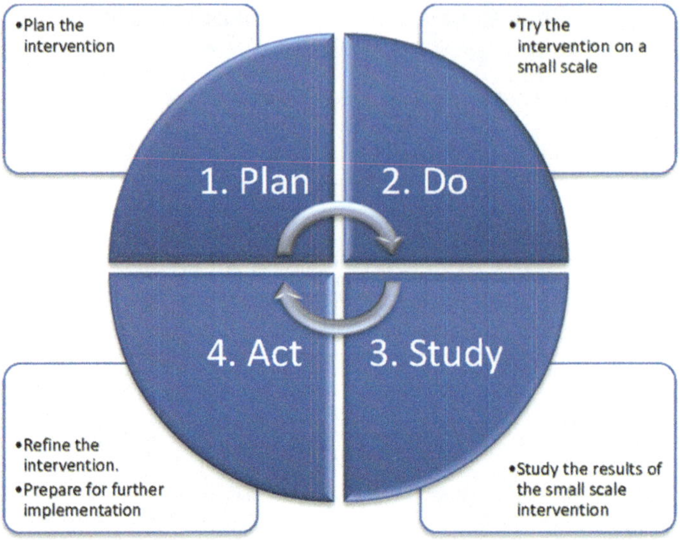

Fig. 5.3 The PDSA cycle (From: http://www.improvingqol.pitt.edu/program-materials/organizational-quick-start-guide. A worksheet for completing the PDSA cycle is available from the IHI: http://www.ihi.org/resources/Pages/Tools/PlanDoStudyActWorksheet.aspx)

about three standard definitions on each side of the mean. Statistical formulas and analyses are applied that can determine if the process is stable or under control (in the desired range) and going in the correct direction. Rules based on changes in consecutive measurements can be used to identify and correct an error in a process and to evaluate the pattern in a process or outcome. Control charts are ideally suited to the visual management approach in Lean Six Sigma and facilitate identification of trends early in their development so that corrective actions can be applied rapidly. The Institute for Healthcare Improvement website has written and video resources on the topic of control charts: http://www.ihi.org/resources/Pages/Tools/RunChart.aspx.

An A3 Report is a Lean method based on the Toyota Production System to guide the BHP through a problem-solving process based on the PDSA cycle and Lean techniques such as current-state analysis, root cause analysis, and measuring changes (Bassuk & Washington, 2013). The A3 Report is used to display and structure problem-solving, a quality improvement project from start to finish. The purpose of the A3 Report is to efficiently display the steps of Lean Six Sigma projects. Commonly used A3 Report steps are (1) problem statement, (2) current state, (3) improvement goal, (4) problem analysis, (5) target future state and measures, (6) implementation plan, (7) verify results, and (8) follow-up.

Performance dashboards are visual management tools designed to monitor processes and outcomes. Dashboards are comprised of easily interpreted graphics such as bar charts, pie charts, or figures that display current performance against strategic goals or improvement targets. Variance from target signals a need for corrective action (Delisle, 2015). Visual management is used to create a snapshot of the current state and trends for key performance indicators (KPIs). The visual cues should be readily understandable to key stakeholders and provide feedback on operational (e.g., BHP productivity, percentage of patients screened for depression) and satisfaction (patient, provider) metrics.

In summary, Lean Six Sigma strategies and techniques begin with tools to document the current state of a process using visual management tools such as the VSM. The emphasis is on identifying VA and NVA components of the process and using problem identification tools such as the root cause analysis fishbone diagram to identify the source of the problem and develop an improvement plan. Project management tools such as the PDSA and A3 Report are used to display all aspects of the project clearly with graphics such as bar charts, pie charts, and control charts to share with the team members. Variation from target goals is identified early in order to develop and test new improvement initiatives rapidly. The goal is to strive for perfection in processes and outcomes.

The BHP is expected to play a leadership role in both promoting Lean Six Sigma in integrated behavioral healthcare settings and to serve as a champion among frontline workers to demonstrate the value of this approach. The BHP will play the role of Lean Six Sigma expert and lead the team is using these techniques to improve efficiency, decrease waste, and improve integrated behavioral health outcomes.

Barriers and Solutions to the Practice of Lean Six Sigma in Integrated Behavioral Health

There are significant barriers to the implementation of Lean Six Sigma for integrated behavioral health. First, behavioral health providers and leaders are not routinely trained and experienced in quality improvement in general and Lean Six Sigma approaches in particular. While Lean Six Sigma approaches are growing in popularity in medical settings, there are relatively few examples specific to integrated behavioral health. One solution to this problem is to study publications on Lean Six Sigma in healthcare and specifically in integrated behavioral health. Excellent textbooks on Lean Six Sigma in healthcare include Dean (2013), Delisle (2015), Graban (2009), Sperl, Placek, and Trewn (2014). Examples of Lean Six Sigma specific to behavioral health include Merlino, Omi, and Bowen (2014), O'Donohue and Maragakis (2016). Another excellent source of content on Lean Six Sigma includes the Institute for Healthcare Improvement (IHI) Online Open School, with many courses on Lean and Six Sigma (http://app.ihi.org/lmsspa/#/6cb1c614-884b-43ef-9abd-d90849f183d4). Finally, there are many online certification courses available. There is no one authorizing body for the Lean or Six Sigma body of knowledge. Accrediting organizations that include the International Association for Six Sigma Certification (IASSC) (http://www.iassc.org) and the Council for Six Sigma Certification (http://www.sixsigmacouncil.org) are available, as are many other education companies, university certificate programs, etc.

Second, Lean Six Sigma is a team-based approach to healthcare improvement, requiring the BHP learner to also master competencies of inter-professional collaboration. Successful implementation of Lean Six Sigma is based upon team-based planning, implementation, and evaluation of the techniques described above. The BHP must obtain buy-in and support from senior leadership in order to launch Lean Six Sigma. Managers and stakeholders from other related departments, such as quality improvement, finance, and health information technology, must contribute to the completion of Lean Six Sigma initiatives. Most importantly, the primary care team, from PCP leader to nursing and allied health staff, to administrative support staff, must be activated and invested in participating on the Lean Six Sigma journey. There are many books and resources on inter-professional teamwork and consultation. An excellent resource for inter-professional education in integrated behavioral health in the American Psychological Association "Curriculum for an Interprofessional Seminar on Integrated Primary Care" (http://www.apa.org/education/grad/curriculum-seminar.aspx).

Third, there is a lack of consensus on what quality measures are necessary for the BCH in integrated behavioral healthcare settings, and measures that are collected are not often utilized in the context of Lean Six Sigma process improvement. Behavioral health providers often view outcomes assessment as too cumbersome given their busy schedules in primary care clinics. Furthermore, these providers are often trained and experienced in using lengthy, traditional psychological assessment approaches that primarily target mental health-related conditions. These providers administer traditional behavioral health measures (e.g., depression, anxiety, and substance use disorder) and neglect the use of measures related to chronic, noncommunicable disease health risks such as nutrition, physical activity, smoking cessation, and medication adherence within their purview. The BHP must include behavioral and medical quality and outcome measures, as well as process measures.

There are two approaches to resolve the problem of quality measurement in integrated behavioral health. The first is to utilize existing primary key performance indicators, typically defined by national and local accreditation organizations. Standardized medical measures such as the CMS Core Quality Measures Collaborative (CMS, 2017) quality metrics (i.e., blood pressure, lipid levels, HbA1c, BMI, and waist circumference) are well-established and often incorporated into VBP contracts. A second approach is to systematically identify integrated behavioral health measures related to the area of performance under review. Goldman, Spaeth-Rublee, Nowels, Ramanuj and Pincus (2016) reviewed quality measures at the interface of behavioral health and primary care. They identified and grouped measures into domains (Table 5.1). BHPs may search for measures from these domains that match the problem under analysis for improvement.

Fourth, VBP approaches to healthcare reimbursement are an emerging, and increasingly common, approach to reimbursement in primary care. However, behavioral health measures are infrequently utilized in value-based pay for performance incentive programs (Stewart, Lareef, Hadley, & Mandell, 2017). Behavioral, patient-reported outcome measures such as the PHQ-9 for depression or process measures

Table 5.1 Quality measures by domains and subdomains by Behavioral Health and General Medical Groupings

Domain	Behavioral health setting measures	Behavioral health subdomain	Measures/ subdomain	General medical setting measures	General medical subdomain	Measures/ subdomain
Screening or diagnostic assessment	64	Screening and follow-up	21	64	Screening and follow-up	18
		Symptomatic/functional ongoing assessment	18		Symptomatic/functional ongoing assessment	32
		Social assessment	0		Social assessment	0
		Substance use assessment	15		Laboratory/imaging ongoing assessment	11
		Suicide risk	5		Other	3
		Blood/urine toxicology	1			
		Other	4			
Evidence-based pharmacotherapy and treatment	77	Selection of medications	14	130	Selection of medications	36
		Medication dosage	0		Medication dosage	3
		Medication adherence	23		Medication adherence	18
		Medication monitoring/ side effects	9		Medication monitoring/ side effects	7
		Medication reconciliation	1		Medication reconciliation	13
		Polypharmacy	9		Polypharmacy	4
		Preventive interventions	0		Preventive-interventions/ immunizations	30
		Psychotherapy	4		Non-pharmacologic treatment/surgery	0
		Brain stimulation treatment	0		Other	19

(continued)

Table 5.1 (continued)

Domain	Behavioral health setting measures	Behavioral health subdomain	Measures/ subdomain	General medical setting measures	General medical subdomain	Measures/ subdomain
		Team-based interventions	1			
		Substance use medications	3			
		Substance use non-pharmacologic treatment	7			
		Other	6			
Patient-centered care	62	Shared decision-making/ patient education	17	67	Shared decision-making/ patient education	20
		Provider-patient communication	8		Provider-patient communication	11
		Patient/family experiences of care	30		Patient/family experiences of care	32
		Recovery	4		Other	4
		Other	3			

From (Goldman et al., 2016)

Table 5.2 Quality targets of phase 1 VBP of the mental health integration program and corresponding fidelity measures

Domain of Collaborative Care	Phase 1 VBP Target	Fidelity Measure
Systematic follow-up	1. Maintain minimum monthly caseload	At least 1 follow-up contact with care manager in each 4-week period
	2. At least 50% caseload receives ≥2 visits to care manager per month	Same as above
Measurement-based care	Not incentivized	At least 1 PHQ-9 assessment in each 4-week period
Stepped care	3. Care coordinators reviewed ≥50% caseload with psychiatrists	At least 1 psychiatric consultation of the case in each 4-week period
	4. Registry documents current psychiatric medication for ≥75% of caseload	Not available[a]

PHQ-9 indicates Patient Health Questionnaire-9, VBP, value-based payment.
[a]Medication data were not available for research.

From (Bao et al., 2017)

such as the HEDIS antidepressant medication measures are not commonly integrated into value-based contracts. In addition, healthcare leaders are often focused on medical measures for value-based care, and do not understand the importance of integrated behavioral interventions necessary to improve medical metrics such as blood pressure, lipids, BMI, and HbA1c.

A recent study by Bao et al. (2017) assessed the effect of a VBP model in improving fidelity and patient outcomes in implementation of the Collaborative Care Model (CCM) of integrated behavioral health. The quality targets in the VBP model are shown in Table 5.2. The study found that a VBP led to significantly improved provider fidelity to practice guidelines and improved depression.

Learning Objectives

The Leans Six Sigma learning objectives (Table 5.3) are comprised of commonly used strategies and techniques of Lean Six Sigma. These competencies are arranged in sequential order that guides the learner from how to assess a problem, initiate an improvement project, establish objective performance goals, use visualization to monitor progress, and implement a rapid improvement event. Ideally, the learner will follow this sequence based on a fictional primary care scenario, or if applicable an actual workplace scenario. For example, a BHP may choose to study the process of a patient attending a primary care clinic to visit their PCP and then participating in a "warm handoff" to the BHP. The VSM evaluation will document each step the patient takes from check-in at the clinic, to the PCP visit, and to the BHP for the warm handoff. The VSM will be used to identify waste or lack of standardization in the process, and a PDSA cycle will be designed to study and improve problems identified. Control charts may be used to monitor key performance indicators for the project, and an A3 Report will be used to share the evaluation results with team members. At any time, a Rapid Improvement Event may be launched to address a performance problem of interest.

Table 5.3 Learning objectives

1. Complete a value stream map and analysis
2. Complete a plan-do-study-act cycle
3. Construct a control chart
4. Create an A3 report
5. Complete a rapid improvement event

Training and Skill Acquisition

The training and skill acquisition activities for each of the core competencies are listed in Table 5.4. Each competency is tied to one of the learning objectives in Table 5.3, but with additional detail added. The learning activities for each competency and approaches to measuring specific competencies are listed. A number of general teaching strategies are applied for each competency. These include (1) reading publications, (2) web searches, (3) quizzes based on content, (4) discussions between learner and instructor, (5) written assignments that demonstrate proficiency at key competencies, (6) role-play presentations to peer learners and/or instructors, and (7) formal presentations to peers and/or instructors. These teaching strategies are applicable to classroom-based, online, or combined hybrid courses given the availability of both asynchronous (e.g., discussion threads) and synchronous (e.g., group webinars) technologies in education.

Measurement and Evaluation

The learning activities are evaluated by written and interactive assignments with well-defined grading rubrics in order to measure and evaluate competencies. The types of assessment include grading of worksheets or papers, class discussion and feedback (in-person or online via discussion board), role-play exercises (in-person or in online group synchronous or asynchronous presentations and feedback), and quizzes. This criterion-based approach to measurement and evaluation is critical in demonstrating competencies in writing exercises, in discussion and feedback, and webinar role-play presentations and feedback reflect the need to demonstrate competencies across these distinct learning modalities.

Examples of measurement and evaluation are included in Appendices A–C. These examples are taken from the ASU College of Health Solutions, Doctor of Behavioral Health online course in quality and performance measurement and improvement. The examples are edited to reduce extraneous detail. Appendix A is a case study scenario of a BHP facing a dilemma in an integrated behavioral health primary care clinic. A case study scenario is necessary for trainees who are not currently working in a primary care clinic setting. This case scenario is used throughout the course as the assignments build upon each other. Appendix B is the instructions

Table 5.4 Lean Six Sigma competencies, learning objectives and activities, and measurement

Competency	Description	Learning objectives	Learning activities	Measurement
Value stream map analysis	Create a value stream map (VSM) with value-added and non-value-added activities, types of waste, and VSM calculations	Complete a VSM analysis Utilize VSM calculations to identify NVA and waste Describe process improvements to increase VA and decrease NVA time	Identify process (real or case study Appendix A) Current-state process map Calculate cycle time; first pass yield; value-added (VA) and non-value-added (NVA) activity; waste; cycle time; wait time; value-adding ratio; and first pass yield	Completed value stream map and calculations Quiz Class role-play presentation Class discussion
Plan-do-study-act (PDSA) cycle	Create a PDSA cycle, ideally based on the QI assignment #1 value stream map assignment	Complete a PDSA worksheet for testing change in an improvement activity	Identify process (real or case study Appendix A) Select measures Define outcome Develop an intervention that you will apply to improve the process and outcome measure Use the "PDSA Worksheet for Testing Change" developed by the IHI	Completed "PDSA Worksheet for Testing Change" worksheet (IHI) Quiz Class role-play presentation Class discussion
Control chart	Create a control chart related to the PDSA	Create a control chart based on PDSA Describe the measure used to create the control chart Create data for control chart based on Rules of Detection to demonstrate trend Describe results of quality improvement activity based on control chart	Select measure from PDSA (process or outcome) Create fictional data for measure Allow about 1/3 of the control chart data points should be "baseline" data before improvement and remaining 2/3 of the data points reflect post-improvement activity Use one or more of the "Rules of Detection in Control Charts" to create trend Complete summary of findings	Completed RVU worksheet for each applicable clinician Quiz Class role-play presentation Class discussion

(continued)

Table 5.4 (continued)

Competency	Description	Learning objectives	Learning activities	Measurement
Rapid improvement event	Complete a Rapid Improvement Event (RIE) and Kaizen problem-solving steps	Design a RIE based on the VSM, PDSA, and control chart assignments with goal of making a process improvement Make a role-play presentation of the RIE Use Action Plan Worksheet to document RIE.	Design a RIE based on the VSM, PDSA, and control chart assignments Assign roles to group members: lead facilitator, process checker, scribe, timekeeper, presenterPresenter follows steps from Kaizen problem-solving process: brainstorm issues and barriers; filter and prioritize issues and barriers; brainstorm solutions; filter and prioritize solutions; develop and implement the action plan using the "Action Plan Worksheet"Describe aspects of the group discussion from the perspective of a team-based approach to quality improvement. Write summary: How did a group approach to planning your RIE add value? What are the benefits of the Kaizen problem-solving process? What are the problems or challenges of using the Kaizen problem-solving process? Complete "action plan template"	Completed RIE worksheet Quiz Class role-play presentation Class discussion
A3 Report	Complete an A3 Report designed to help you "tell the story" of your Lean quality improvement initiative in a logical and visual way to use as a road map for continuous improvement	Complete an A3 Report that combines results of initial VSM, PDSA, and control charts Describe background, problem statement, objective, team, countermeasures Describe results of QI initiative and next steps	Select A3 template (examples provided) Complete: background; problem statement; project/proposal objective; team members; countermeasures; and results. Add future state VSM (in columns 2–3). Add control chart in column 3. Create a basic graphic that reflects an aspect of your project. Complete summary evaluation of results and next steps	A3 Report Quiz Class role-play presentation Class discussion

for the group activity to complete a Rapid Improvement Event (RIE). The group activity is structured as a role-play of a commonly used team-based Lean improvement activity. This assignment is based on an online delivery but can be readily modified to in-person training. Appendix C is a grading rubric for the PDSA group activity.

These examples in Tables A through C are based on an online learning approach but can be easily modified to an in-person training or education approach. These examples were selected to demonstrate measurement and evaluation of strategic approaches to teaching based on completing written assignments, discussions, a group activity, and quiz. For example, online continuing education programs are often asynchronous and do not have the capacity for instructor grading of written assignments. In this case the written assignments can be readily adapted to an online continuing education program by using online quizzes with questions in formats such as true-false, multiple-choice, matching, and fill-in-the blank to test the competency for each component of the written assignment. The group activities can be adopted for online continuing education programs that do not have the capacity for synchronous group meetings by using simulation exercises. These may be constructed in written form such as case studies, in digital video form with recorded group activity vignettes, and by virtual reality programs that present interpersonal scenarios. In each of these examples, the grading rubrics can be readily adapted to online synchronous, asynchronous, or in-person training using principles of effective grading rubrics (Van Leusen, 2013 retrieved from https://teachonline.asu.edu/2013/08/assessments-with-rubrics/#more-2246).

For in-person training programs, the written assignments can also be readily adapted into by having participants complete components of the written exercises alone or in small groups. The group activity exercise is ideal for in-person training and affords the opportunity for students to both demonstrate content mastery but also to practice many professional activities (e.g., completing a pro forma based on existing data, making a role-play presentation of a completed pro forma to peer trainees). Competency may be assessed by observation and ratings based on rubrics for in-person group activity that may be completed by the trainer and may also include peer ratings by peer trainees. Similarly, discussion board assignments may be adapted for in-person training programs by having trainees conduct discussions live that may be observed and rated via rubrics administered by trainers or peer trainees. Creative use of peer trainee ratings may be necessary for large groups of trainees with only one trainer. Even in this case, the trainer can ask each group to have the leader provide a brief, structured summary to the entire group of trainees that the trainee can evaluate for each group. Creative use of mobile phone or tablet apps during training that are designed for trainees to enter responses to questions related to target competencies that create a written record for grading competencies.

Summary

Lean Six Sigma strategies and techniques appear well-suited to meet the emerging demand for improved quality of care, efficiency, outcomes, processes or workflows, and provider work health. All of these areas are part of emerging VBP models that incentivize quality and efficiency over volume. The competencies in this chapter will enable a BHP to implement and evaluate basic Lean Six Sigma strategies and techniques in primary care.

Appendix A: Case Study Scenario

Case Study with Data for Assignment 1: Value Stream Map for Dr. Lynn's Clinic

Instructions: Read this case study carefully. All of the data needed to complete the value stream map formulas are included in the case study. Your job is to create a value stream map of the current state based on this case study.

We met Dr. Lynn last week. She works in a busy urban primary care clinic staffed by an administrative assistant, a scheduler, four PCPs, two nurses, a physician assistant (PA), a medical assistant (MA), and a nutritionist. Dr. Lynn has decided to create a value stream map for process of a patient visit to the PCP, including a warm handoff to the BHP (Dr. Lynn).

Dr. Lynn consulted with all of the staff and identified a basic process map of each step from the time a typical patient first walks in the clinic door until the time the patient walks out of the clinic. Dr. Lynn completed a walk of the process from start to finish to complete the value stream map. All of the times below are based on averages provided by the staff. The times for each process step include the estimated initial first pass yield (PPY) percentage in parenthesis. Dr. Lynn determined the FPY for each process step based on feedback from the team member who is most expert on that step (e.g., administrative assistant for check-in, PCP for PCP interview, etc.).

All patients complete the My Own Health Report (MOHR) as part of their annual physical exam. If one is not on record, the administrative assistant will instruct the patient to complete it in the waiting room after check-in using an office tablet. The physician reviews the MOHR during the patient annual physical exam, but usually not during other visits. Dr. Lynn reviews the MOHR for each new patient. Dr. Lynn will also have the patient complete the full PHQ-9 and GAD-7 if the PHQ-4 that is part of the MOHR is positive. She does this in the session with the patient using a tablet for automatic scoring and feedback. Dr. Lynn may use other rating scales or patient education, self-monitoring, or other forms based on the presenting problem and treatment approach. The clinic has an electronic health record (EHR) system, and all staff enter notes and data for all encounters.

From the time the patient enters the office and approaches the nurses' station, it is one minute. The check-in with the receptionist takes 4 min (FPY, 97%). The patient then waits in the waiting room for 14 min. Then the patient is called in to complete vitals with the PA, which takes 5 min (FPY, 95%). The patient returns to the waiting room and waits for an average of 12 min. Then the patient is called into the examination room for the nurse interview. The nurse interview takes 4 min (FPY, 90%). Then the patient waits in the examination room for an average of 17 min until the PCP arrives for the PCP examination. The PCP examination takes 12 min (FPY, 90%). The PCP then walked the patient to Dr. Lynn's examination room and introduced the patient to Dr. Lynn. This takes 2 min. Dr. Lynn then completes the BHP interview that takes an average of 20 min (FPY, 85%). Upon completion of the BHP interview, the patient returns to the nursing station to check out. Then the patient leaves the office. The clinic is relatively small, so the average time to walk from waiting room to any exam room is 1 min.

Dr. Lynn made several observations during her consultation with the staff and during the process walk. First, Dr. Lynn identified the following high-level process steps:

- Check-in
- Vitals
- Nurses' interview
- Physician exam
- BHP interview
- Checkout

Dr. Lynn also noted the following problems that appeared to contribute to lower first

pass yield (FPY) for each step, that is, problems in each step that resulted in the process step not being completed correctly the first time. During the check-in, the administrative assistant often forgot to ask patients who were there for their annual physical exam to complete the MOHR. During the nursing interview and physician exam, the MOHR results were usually reviewed by the nurse and PCP with the patient. However, the MOHR was not routinely readministered, while the patient was in treatment as a measure of treatment progress and reviewed by the nurse or physician. Dr. Lynn wondered if this should be an area of improvement. During the nursing interview and PCP exam, Dr. Lynn observed that patients were not routinely asked about medication side effects. She thought that this may be an area of quality improvement. During the physician exam, the PCPs typically did not review the MOHR on record for patients who were there for a sick visit.

Each PCP had their own approach to identifying the need for integrated behavioral health referral to Dr. Lynn. Dr. Lynn suspected that the decision-making processes for identifying and referring patients to her were not consistent between the PCPs and may be an area of improvement. Dr. Lynn also observed that sometimes patients were not clear why they were referred to see her in the warm handoff. Patients reported not being clear on her role and purpose of the referral. Dr. Lynn identified the need for improved patient information on her service, and perhaps a script for PCPs would be a potential area of improvement. During her own patient visits, Dr. Lynn noticed that she often spent too much time going over the MOHR and other rating scales she administered, leaving her feeling rushed to transition to the treatment planning, advising and assisting the patient to leave with a clear and agreed-upon plan of action for behavioral issues. Dr. Lynn reviewed the wait times between each process step and did not think that they were excessive for a busy clinic. However, she realized that she had not reviewed the clinic patient satisfaction data available on this topic. In addition, Dr. Lynn noted that while there were some magazines in the waiting room, they were older, and only a few subscriptions were available. She thought that having magazines in the exam rooms may also be helpful, and she wondered if a TV added to the waiting room would be helpful.

Appendix B: Group Activity #2 – Rapid Improvement Event

Use the discussion group thread for your group to contact your group members and schedule a meeting (teleconference, skype, etc.). For this group activity, you will practice a group Rapid Improvement Event.

1. Carefully read "Facilitating Rapid Improvements" Chap. 9 from "*Executing Lean Improvements*" by Delisle (2015). Each group member will prepare a Rapid Improvement Event (RIE) based on your quality improvement project for this class (the VSM, PDSA, and control chart).
2. Assign team roles to each member based on the roles under "Facilitation Guidelines" on page 158 (you may swap roles as each group member takes turns as "presenter"):

   Lead facilitator, process checker, scribe, timekeeper, and presenter

3. *Each presenter will choose a technique from each of the five steps of the "Kaizen problem-solving process"*

   Step 1. Brainstorm issues and barriers.
   Step 2. Filter and prioritize issues and barriers.
   Step 3. Brainstorm solutions.
   Step 4. Filter and prioritize solutions.
   Step 5. Develop and implement the action plan using the "Action Plan Worksheet."

   Note that each presenter will choose one of the multiple techniques listed under Steps 1–5 above. Also note that a number of techniques are designed for an in-person rather than telephonic meeting. You may choose an in-person technique provided that you can modify it for a telephonic meeting.

4. *Each member will take a turn making their presentation based on the Kaizen problem-solving process.* Note: Be brief, and modify each presentation so that you will complete your presentation and all steps in about 20 min. A real Kaizen problem-solving exercise would take at least 1 hour or more. For this assignment, I am interested in your ability to practice each technique briefly, but not to spend so much time that the duration of your group meeting is excessive.

I recommend that the group agree on a time limit for each presentation and that the "timekeeper" announce in 5-min increments the time remaining.

5. *Complete a final group thread posting. Note: You do not need to post a substantive reply for this assignment.* The final group thread posting for each group member should include each of the following:

   (a) Describe aspects of the group discussion from the perspective of a team-based approach to quality improvement. How did a group approach to planning your RIE add value? What are the benefits of the Kaizen problem-solving process? What are the problems or challenges of using the Kaizen problem-solving process?
   (b) Post your "action plan template." You can post as a summary narrative in the group thread; you do not need to use a table format as used in book example.

Appendix C: Group Activity PDSA Grading Rubric

PDSA group activity grading rubric

Category	Excellent 1	Good 0.75	Fair 0.50	Poor 0.25
Brief description of PDSA	Contains clear and concise description that includes aim, plan, do, and study	Contains general description that includes aim, plan, do, and study	Contains fair description that does not clearly include aim, plan, do, and study	Contains poor description that does not clearly include aim, plan, do, and study
Brief description of control chart	Contains clear and concise description of measure selected for control chart	Contains general description of measure selected for control chart	Contains fair description of measure selected for control chart	Contains poor description of measure selected for control chart
Brief description of your presentation and discussion	Contains clear and concise description of your experience in presenting and discussing your PDSA/control chart. Clear description of how feedback influenced your plan for assignment	Contains general description of your experience in presenting and discussing your PDSA/control chart. General description of how feedback influenced your plan for assignment	Contains fair description of your experience in presenting and discussing your PDSA/control chart. Not clear how feedback influenced your plan for assignment	Contains poor and concise description of your experience in presenting and discussing your PDSA/control chart. Not stated how feedback influence your plan for assignment
Clarity and mechanics	Excellent. No grammar or spelling errors. Excellent organization	Good. One grammar or spelling error. Good organization	Fair. More than one grammar or spelling error. Fair organization	Poor. More than one grammar or spelling error. Poor organization

References

Bao, Y., McGuire, T., Chan, Y., Eggman, A., Ryan, A. M., Bruce, M. L., et al. (2017). Value-based payment in implementing evidence-based care: The mental health integration program in Washington State. *American Journal of Managed Care, 23*(1), 48–53.

Bassuk, J., & Washington, I. (2013). The A3 problem solving report: A 10-step scientific method to execute performance improvements in an academic research vivarium. *PLoS ONE, 8*(10), e76833. https://doi.org/10.1371/journal.pone.0078633.

Berwick, D., Nolan, T., & Whittington, J. (2008). The triple aim: Care, health, and cost. *Health Affairs, 27*(3), 759–769. https://doi.org/10.1377/hlthaff.27.3.759.

Blumenthal, D., & McGinnis, J. (2015). Measuring vital signs: And IOM report on core metrics for health and health care progress. *JAMA, 313*(19), 1901–1902. https://doi.org/10.1001/jama.2015.4862.

Bodenheimer, T., & Sinsky, C. (2014). From triple to quadruple aim: Care of the patient requires care of the provider. *Annals of Family Medicine, 12*, 573–576. https://doi.org/10.1370/afm.1713.

Chalice, R. (2007). *Improving healthcare using Toyota lean production methods* (2nd ed.). Milwaukee, WI: ASO Quality.

CMS Core Measures: Quality Measures. Retrieved on July 20, 2017 from https://www.cms.gov/Medicare/Quality-Initiatives-Patient-Assessment-Instruments/QualityMeasures/Core-Measures.html

Dean, M. (2013). *Lean healthcare deployment and sustainability*. New York: McGraw Hill.

Deblois, S., & Lepanto, L. (2016). Lean and six sigma in acute care: A systematic review. *International Journal of Healthcare Quality Assurance, 29*(2), 192–208. https://doi.org/10.1108/JHCQA-05-2014-0058.

Delisle, D. (2015). *Executing lean improvements: A practical guide with real-world healthcare case studies*. Milwaukee: ASQ Quality.

Delisle, D. (2016). *Executing lean improvements: a practical guide with real-world healthcare case studies*. Milwaukee, WI: ASQ Quality Press.

Glasgow, J., Scott-Caziewell, J., & Kaboli, P. (2010). Guiding inpatient quality improvement: A systematic review of Lean and Six Sigma. *Joint Commission Journal on Quality and Patient Safety, 36*(12), 544–540.

Goldman, M., Spaeth-Rublee, B., Nowels, A., Ramanuj, P., & Pincus, H. (2016). Quality measures at the interface of behavioral health and primary care. *Current Psychiatry Reports, 18*, 39. https://doi.org/10.1007/s11920-016-0671-8.

Graban, M. (2009). *Lean hospitals: Improving quality, safety, and employee satisfaction*. New York: CRC.

Institute of Medicine. (2001). *Crossing the quality Chasm: A new health system for the twenty-first century*. Washington, DC: National Academies.

Joint Commission on the Accreditation of Healthcare Organizations. (2006). *Doing more with less: Lean thinking and patient safety in health care*. Oakbrook, IL: Joint Commission on the Accreditation of Healthcare Organizations.

Kessler, R. (2012). Effects on mental health treatment initiation when mental health services are incorporated into primary care practice. *Journal of the American Board of Family Medicine, 25*(2), 255–259.

Kessler, R., Miller, B., Kelly, M., Graham, D., Kennedy, A., Littenberg, B., et al. (2014). Mental health, substance abuse, and health behavior services in patient-centered medical homes. *Journal of the American Board of Family Medicine, 27*(5), 637–644.

Merlino, J., Omi, J., & Bowen, J. (2014). *Lean behavioral health: The Kings County Hospital story*. New York: Oxford University Press.

Napier, R. (2017). *Value stream map for diabetes clinic patient visit*. Classroom assignment from Arizona State University, Doctor of Behavioral Health class: IBC 714 Quality and Performance Measurement, Improvement, and Incentives, Fall A.

O'Donohue, W., & Maragakis, A. (Eds.). (2016). *Quality improvement in behavioral health*. AG Switzerland: Springer.

Robinson, P., & Reiter, J. (2016). *Behavioral consultation and primary care: A guide to integrating services* (2nd ed.). New York: Springer.

Sperl, T., Placek, R., & Trewn, J. (2014). *Practical Lean Six Sigma for healthcare: Using the A3 and lean thinking to improve operational performance in hospitals, clinics and physician group practices*. Chelsea, MI: MCD Media.

Stewart, R., Lareef, I., Hadley, R., & Mandell, D. (2017). Can we pay for performance in behavioral health care? *Psychiatric Services, 68*, 2.

Thomas-Henkel, C., Hamblin, A., & Hendricks, T. (2015, November). *Supporting a culture of health for high-need, high-cost populations: Opportunities to improve models of care for people with complex needs*. The Robert Wood Johnson Foundation and the Center for Health Care Strategies.

Womack, J., & Jones, D. (2003). *Lean thinking*. New York: Free Press.

Chapter 6
BHP Performance on Medical Teams

Lesley Manson

Chapter overview	
Domains	*Evidence-based health care* *Move behavioral health (BH) from carve out to carve in as an integral part of comprehensive, integrated health-care delivery* *Health-care delivery improvements and efficiencies* *Measuring levels of integrated health care* *Integrated health-care workforce training*
Key points	*Unique and complimentary roles with other providers, models of team-based care, the Interprofessional Education Collaborative (IPEC®) Core Competencies for Interprofessional Collaborative Practice* (2016), *team-based decision-making, intervention, and treatment planning; communication and collaboration on medical teams; team-based clinical practice; team-based assessment and activities to enhance clinical care; measuring team-based care*
Foundational knowledge and skills	*Ability to design, deliver, and evaluate behavioral health provider performance as a member of a health-care team.*
Student learning objectives (SLOs)	*1) Describe the essential features of team-based communication and collaboration facilitating practice management and patient outcomes* *2) Identify the individual roles and responsibilities of the integrated primary care team member related to patient and team-based care* *3) Identify the key competencies of the integrated behavioral health provider within the medical team or clarify team roles and responsibilities to optimize efficiency, outcomes, and accountability*
Instructional strategies	*Lecture, discussion, video/media, assigned readings, role-play, coaching, and presentations*
Evaluating learning	*Quizzes, written assignments, grading discussions, presentations, and graded demonstrations/role-plays*

L. Manson (✉)
Integrated Behavioral Health Programs, College of Health Solutions,
Arizona State University, Phoenix, AZ, USA
e-mail: lesley.manson@asu.edu

C. R. Macchi, R. Kessler (eds.), *Training to Deliver Integrated Care*,
https://doi.org/10.1007/978-3-319-78850-0_6

Historical/Traditional Approaches to Training Issues

Historically, approaches to traditional training have been segregated and siloed based upon their professional guild (e.g., medicine, psychology, social work). This segregated process is reinforced by accreditation, regulatory bodies, and licensure boards. It does not provide foundational skills in team based care to health-care professionals to understand team-based roles and seamlessly operate in teams (Doumouras, Keshet, Nathens, Ahmed, & Hicks, 2014; Landman, Aannestad, Smoldt, & Cortese, 2014). Both the National Academy of Medicine (formerly known as the Institute of Medicine (IOM)) and the Agency for Healthcare Research and Quality (AHRQ) suggest patient safety and care coordination can be enhanced by training in teamwork (Mitchell et al., 2012). The current movement toward team-based health care suggests that we promote a broader adoption of team-based care models, encourage value-based reimbursement models, and build team-based education of health professionals (Landman et al., 2014).

Key Conceptual and Operational Shifts

The IOM reports on health-care quality in the USA (*To err is human: Building a safer health system*, 1999 and *Crossing the quality chasm: A new health system for the twenty-first century*, 2001) were pivotal in the shift toward an integrated model of team-based health-care design. These comprehensive reports highlighted the problems and limitations of health care noting broad overuse of medical resources, underuse of known benefits and needed resources, misuse of health-care resources and treatments, and medical errors. The final recommendations presented a new comprehensive framework for health-care delivery provided in a team-based format, inclusive of behavioral/mental health professionals, and focused on six dimensions of health care: patient safety, care effectiveness, patient-centeredness, timeliness, care efficiency, and equity. This recommended shift provided crucial support of federal health-care and payment reform to align with team-based services and integrated care efforts. Health-care entities, inclusive of workforce training and degree programs, began to shift from their siloed training toward a collaborative, team-based model.

Foundational, collaborative, coordinated team-based care skills are being incorporated into health education and clinical training programs across all disciplines participating in team-based care. Skills focus on interprofessional competencies (Interprofessional Education Collaborative (IPEC), 2011, 2016), such as the seven C's of teamwork (i.e., coordination, collaboration, communication, conflict, cognition, coaching, and cooperation; Salas, Shuffler, Thayer, Bedwell, & Lazzara, 2015) and the core principles (i.e., shared goals, clear roles, mutual trust, effective communication, and measurable processes and outcomes; IOM, 2006; Mitchell et al., 2012). Health-care professionals providing team-based care have demonstrated improved patient health outcomes and satisfaction while controlling health-care delivery costs (Cortese & Smoldt, 2013; Feachem, Sekhri, & White, 2002; Mills, 2013).

Practitioner Performance Barriers to Team-Based Integration

It is important for trainers to utilize interprofessional teams to identify barriers and strategies toward success. The most notable barriers include inadequate training for effective teamwork, limited time and resources to build teams and trust, clash of cultures, lack of structure to support team-based care in daily workflows and decision-making, and insufficient feedback on team functioning and goals (Mitchell et al.; 2012).

Identifying facilitators and barriers to implementing a redesigned team-based health-care model will simplify effort. Trainers may wish to bring interprofessional groups and teams together to identify specific people and tools that facilitate team-based care success. Facilitators may include champions on the teams that advocate for team-based care and decision-making, shared medical records and communication processes, and shared work spaces. The core principles of effective teams are demonstrated to include shared goals, clear roles, mutual trust, effective communication, and measureable processes and outcomes (IOM, 2006; Mitchell et al., 2012). Health-care sites vary in the opportunities and required elements to support team-based functioning. Trainers may wish to evaluate health-care sites for team-based care opportunities and readiness or empower their learners toward a team-based focus.

Team-Based Training or Skill Acquisition

The foundational knowledge for team-based training is interprofessional education (IPEC, 2011, 2016). To incorporate IPE into training programs requires bridging education in IPE competencies (values and ethics for interprofessional practice, roles and responsibilities, interprofessional communication, teams and teamwork) with practical applications in practice (see Table 6.1). Team-based practice and application in team scenarios is best accomplished in interprofessional groups and teams. In addition, instructors are encouraged to utilize learning tools such as foundational knowledge checks (quizzes, comprehension scenarios), role-plays, team shadowing, skill observation, and feedback (applying skill observation to assessment and feedback). Through role-plays the learner can practice the competencies in a non-threatening manner, progress to shadowing teams who apply such skills, apply skills in teams, and then observe teams and identify specific skills for applied feedback. Learners progressing through this cycle receive foundational, team-based workforce training (see Fig. 6.1).

Table 6.1 IPE Competencies and training application

IPE Competency	Training application/key performance indicators	Competency	Sub-competency
values and ethics (VE)	Acknowledge a person's right to make choices, to hold views, and to take actions based on personal values and beliefs Acknowledges the patient and their supports as central to the health-care team Demonstrate respect to all team members Respects and considers culture and diversity in treatment planning and communication Shows respect for other health-care team member values and ethics, person-centered considerations, and learns from others to ensure a balanced approach to ethical decision-making Understands and demonstrates competency of one's professional ethics and values	Maintains a climate of mutual respect and shared values	VE1. Place interests of patients and populations at the center of interprofessional health-care delivery and population health programs and policies, with the goal of promoting health and health equity across the life span VE2. Respect the dignity and privacy of patients while maintaining confidentiality in the delivery of team-based care VE3. Embrace the cultural diversity and individual differences that characterize patients, populations, and the health team VE4. Respect the unique cultures, values, roles/responsibilities, and expertise of other health professions and the impact these factors can have on health outcomes VE5. Work in cooperation with those who receive care, those who provide care, and others who contribute to or support the delivery of prevention and health services and programs VE6. Develop a trusting relationship with patients, families, and other team members VE7. Demonstrate high standards of ethical conduct and quality of care in contributions to team-based care VE8. Manage ethical dilemmas specific to interprofessional patient-/population-centered care situations VE9. Act with honesty and integrity in relationships with patients, families, communities, and other team members VE10. Maintain competence in one's own profession appropriate to scope of practice

Roles and responsibilities (RR)	Verbalizes one's role and responsibilities to patients, community, supports, and the health-care team. Creates flyers to communicate essential roles and responsibilities of the health-care team Acknowledges the scope of practice Builds community partnerships for improve health access and outcomes Works collaboratively within the health-care team to build shared treatment plans, interventions, and care Engages in team/team-based development, building, and learning/research activities Communicates how professionals in health and other fields can collaborate and integrate clinical care and public health interventions to optimize population health Builds population health programs identifying roles and responsibilities and shared responsibilities	Assesses and addresses the health-care needs of patients and promotes and advances the health of populations through knowledge of one's own role and those of the other health-care team members/professionals	RR1. Communicate one's roles and responsibilities clearly to patients, families, community members, and other professionals. RR2. Recognize one's limitations in skills, knowledge, and abilities RR3. Engage diverse professionals who complement one's own professional expertise, as well as associated resources, to develop strategies to meet specific health and health-care needs of patients and populations RR4. Explain the roles and responsibilities of other providers and how the team works together to provide care, promote health, and prevent disease RR5. Use the full scope of knowledge, skills, and abilities of professionals from health and other fields to provide care that is safe, timely, efficient, effective, and equitable RR6. Communicate with team members to clarify each member's responsibility in executing components of a treatment plan or public health intervention RR7. Forge interdependent relationships with other professions within and outside of the health system to improve care and advance learning RR8. Engage in continuous professional and interprofessional development to enhance team performance and collaboration RR9. Use unique and complementary abilities of all members of the team to optimize health and patient care RR10. Describe how professionals in health and other fields can collaborate and integrate clinical care and public health interventions to optimize population health

(continued)

Table 6.1 (continued)

IPE Competency	Training application/key performance indicators	Competency	Sub-competency
Communication (CC)	Communicates verbally and nonverbally, utilizing electronic health records, to ensure team-based care Uses person-centered communication and health and numeracy literacy to ensure communication is appropriate and understandable to patients, supports, and community Uses SBAR, speaker listener techniques, MI, and other evidence-based communication approaches in teams and with patients, supports, and community Ensures all team members feel comfortable, supported, and are active in huddles and care processes Provides relevant, timely, and appropriate feedback to team members as needed Manages team conflict and feedback Understands, recognizes, manages, and communicates about power elements in teams, patient care, and related to culture Ensures to communicate and advocate for team-based policies and procedures for population health	Communication supports a team-based approach to the promotion and maintenance of health and prevention and treatment of disease Communicates with patients, families, communities, and other team members in a responsive and responsible manner	CC1. Choose effective communication tools and techniques, including information systems and communication technologies, to facilitate discussions and interactions that enhance team function CC2. Communicate information with patients, families, community members, and health team members in a form that is understandable, avoiding discipline-specific terminology when possible CC3. Express one's knowledge and opinions to team members involved in patient care and population health improvement with confidence, clarity, and respect, working to ensure common understanding of information, treatment, care decisions, and population health programs and policies CC4. Listen actively and encourage ideas and opinions of other team members CC5. Give timely, sensitive, instructive feedback to others about their performance on the team, responding respectfully as a team member to feedback from others CC6. Use respectful language appropriate for a given difficult situation, crucial conversation, or conflict CC7. Recognize how one's own uniqueness (experience level, expertise, culture, power, and hierarchy within the health team) contributes to effective communication, conflict resolution, and positive interprofessional working relationships CC8. Communicate the importance of teamwork in patient-centered care and population health programs and policies

Teams and teamwork (TT)	Team decision-making Team treatment planning Huddles Care appointments focusing on team goals Evaluating evidence-based approaches to care through a team lens Acknowledging the patient as an essential team member Sharing accountability through assessing patients through team lens and priorities Team process improvement projects	Applies relationship-building values and the principles of team dynamics to perform effectively within the team Applies these values and principles to plan, deliver, and evaluate patient/population-centered care and population health programs and policies which are safe, timely, efficient, effective, and equitable	TT1. Describe the process of team development and the roles and practices of effective teams TT2. Develop consensus on the ethical principles to guide all aspects of team work TT3. Engage health and other professionals in shared patient-centered and population-focused problem-solving TT4. Integrate the knowledge and experience of health and other professions to inform health and care decisions, while respecting patient and community values and priorities/preferences for care TT5. Apply leadership practices that support collaborative practice and team effectiveness TT6. Engage self and others to constructively manage disagreements about values, roles, goals, and actions that arise among health and other professionals and with patients, families, and community members TT7. Share accountability with other professions, patients, and communities for outcomes relevant to prevention and health care TT8. Reflect on individual and team performance for individual, as well as team, performance improvement TT9. Use process improvement to increase effectiveness of interprofessional teamwork and team-based services, programs, and policies TT10. Use available evidence to inform effective teamwork and team-based practices TT11. Perform effectively on teams and in different team roles in a variety of settings

IPEC (2016). Core Competencies for Interprofessional Collaborative Practice: Report of an Expert Panel. Washington, DC. Retrieved from: https://ipecollaborative.org/uploads/IPEC-Core-Competencies.pdf

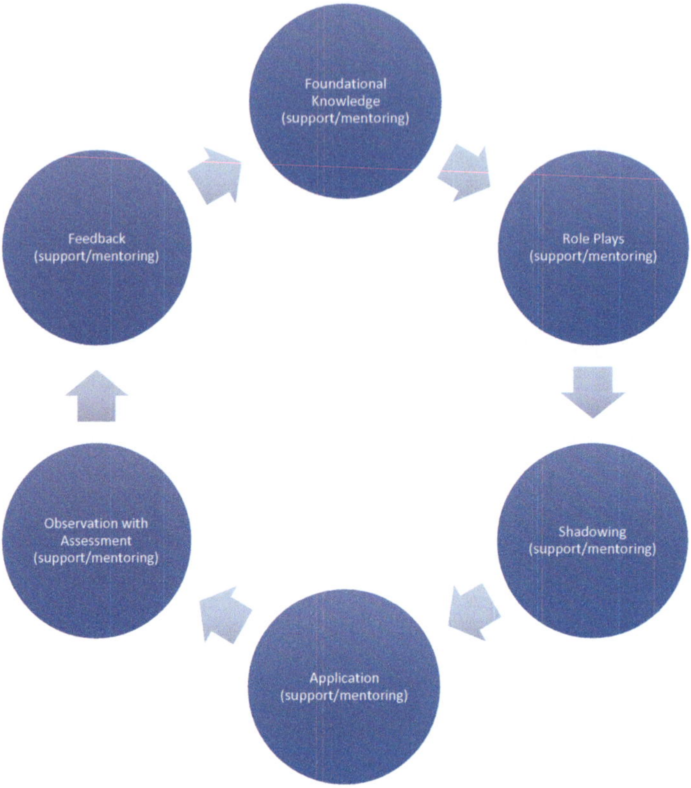

Fig. 6.1 Workforce training cycle

Training Priorities and Resources for Team-Based Care

Evidence-based resources exist to support a successful team-based training program (see Table 6.2) (Agency for Healthcare Research and Quality, 2014; Institute for Healthcare Improvement (2016a, b, c); Interprofessional Education Collaborative Expert Panel, 2011). Training programs may supplement their learning materials with the online curricula and training resources found on these websites. Further, the workforce training cycle (see Fig. 6.1) identifies learning, role-plays, and comparisons that provide traditional and team-based clinical case examples to assist learners identify team-based communication, interventions, roles and responsibilities, decision-making, shared care planning, and care coordination opportunities. There are also assessments from these team-based curricula.

Table 6.2 Team-based resources

Resource	Training application	Website
Team STEPPS	An evidence-based teamwork system to improve communication and teamwork skills among health-care professionals A source for ready-to-use materials and a training curriculum to successfully integrate teamwork principles into all areas of your health-care system	https://www.ahrq.gov/teamstepps/about-teamstepps/index.html
Teamlet model (Bodenheimer & Laing, 2007; Bodenheimer, 2008)	The teamlet model is associated with better patient and staff experience, improved clinical quality measures, and reduced health-care costs	https://cepc.ucsf.edu/teamlets
Train-the-Trainer Interprofessional Faculty Development Program (T3-IFDP)	Evidence-based faculty development program for health professional faculty and clinicians working with interprofessional (IP) and collaborative practice (IPCP) initiatives who want to enhance their leadership skills and capabilities to lead IP efforts in their organizations. Provides coaching and evaluations	https://nexusipe.org/t3-train-trainer-faculty-development-program-interprofessional-education-faculty-development
The American Interprofessional Health Collaborative (AIHC)	AIHC transcends boundaries to transform learning, policies, practices, and scholarship toward an improved system of health and wellness for individual patients, communities, and populations. It believes educating those entrusted with the health of individuals, communities, and populations to value and respect each other's unique expertise and skills, and to work together is fundamental to care that is effective, safe, of high quality, and efficient in terms of cost, resources, and time. The AIHC Interprofessional webinar series offers a forum for leaders who are committed to systems transformation through interprofessional collaboration and learning	https://aihc-us.org/
Agency for Healthcare Research and Quality (AHRQ)	AHRQ's mission is to produce evidence to make health care safer, higher quality, more accessible, equitable, and affordable and to work within the US Department of Health and Human Services and with other partners to make sure that the evidence is understood and used Website includes curricula for team building, research, tools, data, and funding opportunities	https://www.ahrq.gov/

(continued)

Table 6.2 (continued)

Resource	Training application	Website
Institute for Healthcare Improvement (IHI)	The mission of IHI is to improve the health of individuals and populations. To advance their mission, IHI's work is focused in five key areas of improving capability, person- and family-centered care, and patient safety and improving quality, cost, and value; triple aim for populations	http://www.ihi.org
University of Washington's advancing integrated mental health solutions	Learn how to implement collaborative care, a specific type of integrated care developed at the University of Washington The University of Washington's AIMS Center develops, tests, and helps implement collaborative care, an evidence-based integrated care model that brings high-quality mental health care to familiar settings AIMS provides coaching and implementation support, research collaborations, and education and workforce development.	https://aims.uw.edu/
Substance Abuse and Mental Health Services Administration (SAMHSA) – Health Resources and Services Administration (HRSA) Center for Integrated Health Solutions	Access to tools, integrated care models, workforce training information, financing, clinical practice guides, operations and administration information, and best practice information for health and wellness	https://www.integration.samhsa.gov/about-us/what-is-integrated-care
National Center for Interprofessional practice and education (IPEC National Center)	IPEC National Center offers and supports evaluation, research, data, and evidence that ignites the field of interprofessional practice and education and leads to better care, added value, and healthier communities	https://nexusipe.org/

Measurement of Team-Based Performance Skills and Outcomes

Successful training programs generate successful learning but also provide mentoring, support, and quality feedback. In addition, an instructor will develop achievable goals that set clear targets for measurement. Essential tools include, rubrics, training guides, established curricula learning checks, assessments, and competency tools. Research and best practice supports the use of the following tools for team-based skill and performance measurement (see Table 6.3) (Agency for Healthcare Research and Quality, 2014; Institute for Healthcare Improvement (2016a, b, c); Interprofessional Education Collaborative Expert Panel, 2011). In addition, training programs may wish to utilize other outcome assessments such as those listed in Table 6.3. They may include improved patient and team satisfaction, patient outcomes, reduced medical errors, enhanced patient engagement and adherence, decreased no-show rates, number of completed team-based integrated treatment plans, review of documentation identifying team-based communication and shared responsibility, coordination of care, and improved patient understanding of treatment plans, interventions, and diagnosis. Instructors may wish to create unique assessment tools for these evaluations, compare results to national statistics, and/or utilize national assessments such as National Center for Quality Assurance patient-centered medical home evaluations, clinician, and group survey comparative data for health plans (CGCAHPS) national survey data.

Example Template for Developing a Training Program

It is essential for trainers to consider the priorities in team-based skill development to optimize care delivery (Agency for Healthcare Research and Quality, 2014; Institute for Healthcare Improvement (2016a, b, c); Interprofessional Education Collaborative Expert Panel, 2011). Refocusing behavioral health providers to broaden from a siloed practice approach to a team-based approach takes skill development. Trainers may wish to create opportunities for the behavioral health provider to demonstrate each of the skills in Table 6.3 and utilize the resources listed to generate rubrics and measured evaluations. Trainers must be creative in highlighting examples from general traditional care and challenging the learner to take a team-based approach. For example, the learner must be able to identify team-based approaches to address mood, depression, attention deficit, anxiety, sleep, and weight concerns in a team-based medical setting as noted in Table 6.4. This redesign must include the evaluation of the skills noted above through an integrated team-based lens (addressing medical and behavioral care needs). Through effective team-based skill development, behavioral health providers will be ready for the challenge of working on medical care teams and meeting the quadruple aims of health care.

Table 6.3 Team-based skill and performance measurement and training priorities

Skill/priorities	Training application	Resource
Huddles	Huddle competency tool was developed to assist organizations with monitoring and evaluating huddle success. The tool can be adapted to the structure and needs of each health-care team huddle	See sample in book on page X
Shared communication: SBAR	The SBAR competency tool was developed to assist organizations with monitoring and evaluating the use of SBAR communication technique	See sample in book on page X
Team skills: Collaborative Practice Assessment Tool (CPAT)	CPAT was developed to assess levels of collaboration intended to assist clinical teams in identifying strengths and weaknesses in their collaborative practice thereby providing opportunities for focused educational interventions The Collaborative Practice Assessment Tool (CPAT) is a 57-item tool with a 7-point scale that assesses collaborative practice. The tool has eight subscales: mission, meaningful purpose and goals, general relationships, team leadership, general role, responsibilities and autonomy, communication and information exchange, community linkages and coordination of care, decision-making and conflict management, and patient involvement	https://nexusipe.org/informing/resource-center/cpat-collaborative-practice-assessment-tool
Team skills: Assessment for Collaborative Environments (ACE)	The ACE-15 was designed to help faculty and administrators conduct a rapid assessment of the quality of interprofessional teamwork in clinical sites Results can be used as a guide for placing learners (students, residents) in positive teaching environments in which interprofessional collaboration is being modeled. This 15-item, self-report survey is appropriate for a broad array of health professionals working in a variety of clinical sites. A validity study including 192 health-care professionals from 17 clinical professions demonstrated good factor structure and internal reliability. ACE-15 scores significantly related to a separate measure of team cohesion	https://nexusipe.org/advancing/assessment-evaluation/assessment-collaborative-environments-ace-15

IPEC competency: National Center for IPEC	Interprofessional education and competency is an important skill. The resource center for team-based evaluation and assessment tools may be beneficial for identifying evaluation, assessment tools, and metrics surrounding IPEC	https://nexusipe.org/informing/resource-center
Warm handoff	Warm handoffs are an essential skill for BHP on medical teams. Trainers may wish to build assessment and metrics focused around timing, brevity, accessibility, communication, documentation, and shared planning	
Shared decision-making	BHPs must demonstrate the ability to communicate with team members, patients, and families. This communication may be best assessed through observation or review of documentation related. BHPs must be efficient at documenting shared decision-making and/or using shared decision-making tools. Shared decision-making tools may be obtaining through AHRQ	https://www.ahrq.gov/professionals/education/curriculum-tools/shareddecisionmaking/index.html
Shared treatment plans	Developing shared treatment plans is essential. BHPs must demonstrate the ability to develop treatment plans which incorporate interprofessional goals, monitoring of progress, and assessment	https://nexusipe.org/informing/resource-center/developing-integrated-plan-care
Interprofessional psychoeducation and training	An essential role of a BHP on medical teams is as an educator. Trainers may wish to evaluate BHPs on delivery of psychoeducation and trainings on mental and behavioral health topics, comorbidities, care paths, and behavioral medicine topics. In addition, trainers may also wish to emphasize a BHPs role to deliver such education and training in community settings to patients, families, and supports using appropriate health literacy	

(continued)

Table 6.3 (continued)

Skill/priorities	Training application	Resource
Medical team enhancement of outcomes	Evaluation of BHPs on medical teams may also be conducted through a secondary approach of comparison pre-and post-evaluation of national quality metric data such as patient satisfaction, health (HEDIS), National Quality Forum (NQF), or Patient- Centered Medical Home (PCMH) data	1. Patient satisfaction: https://www.ahrq.gov/cahps/surveys-guidance/cg/index.html 2. HEDIS: http://www.ncqa.org/hedis-quality-measurement 3. NQF: https://www.qualityforum.org/Measures_Reports_Tools.aspx 4. PCMH: http://www.ncqa.org/programs/recognition/practices/patient-centered-medical-home-pcmh
Roles and responsibilities	It is the responsibility of each team member to effectively communicate and understand the scope of practice, roles, and responsibilities of each team member. BHPs must practice effectively describing their own roles in team-based care as well as the other members of the health-care team and how they interact, collaborate, and communicate	https://nexusipe.org/informing/resource-center/roles-and-responsibilities-it-takes-team

Table 6.4 Depression treatment team-based skill and performance training plan examples

Skill/Priorities	Training Application
Huddles	Role-play identifying, treating, or assessing depression in huddles
Interprofessional psychoeducation and training	Role-play providing depression management psychoeducation to patients, families, and communities at an appropriate literacy level. Practice psychoeducation and training for medical team members which highlights a team-based, behavioral medicine approach to depression management
IPEC competency: National Center for IPEC	Ensure the BHP can communicate how each of the areas of IPEC competency pertains to team-based treatment of depression in a medical center
Medical team enhancement of outcomes	Ensure the BHP can identify specific outcome measurements for depression in medical settings
Roles and responsibilities	Role-play communication of how each team member will work together to treat depression with the patient
Shared communication: SBAR	Role-play communication to another team member about a patient's depression utilizing SBAR
Shared decision-making	Ensure the BHP demonstrates using a shared decision-making tool working with patients to solidify self-management skills and care plans
Shared treatment plans	Review the BHP's treatment plan to ensure incorporation of interprofessional goals, monitoring of progress, and assessment
Warm handoff	Practice brief interventions for depression management

Conclusion

Through redesigning curricula to meet the demands of integrated team-based care, we will successfully prepare our behavioral health workforce to meet the quadruple aims of health care. As behavioral health providers develop these unique multidisciplinary skills, they will demonstrate their worth, role, and responsibility on the integrated medical team.

References

Agency for Healthcare Research and Quality. (2014). *Teamwork perceptions questionnaire (T-TPQ): Team STEPPS instructor manual*. Retrieved from http://www.ahrq.gov/teamstepps/instructor/reference/teampercept.html

Bodenheimer, T. (2008). Coordinating Care — A Perilous Journey through the Health Care System. The New England Journal of Medicine, 358(10), 1064–1071. https://doi.org/10.1056/NEJMhpr0706165.

Bodenheimer T, Laing BY (2007). The Teamlet Model of Primary Care. *Annals of Family Medicine, 5*(5), 457–461.

Cortese, D. A. & Smoldt, R. K. (2013). *A roadmap to high-value healthcare delivery*. Retrieved from http://healthcaretransformationinstitute.org/sites/default/files/HVHC_070612%20final.pdf

Doumouras, A. G., Keshet, I., Nathens, A. B., Ahmed, N., & Hicks, C. M.. (2014, June). (TNT-2): The development, piloting and multilevel assessment of a simulation-based, interprofessional curriculum for team-based trauma resuscitation. *Annuals of Surgery, 259*(6), 1041–53. Doi: https://doi.org/10.1097/SLA.0000000000000595.

Feachem, R. G., Sekhri, N. K., & White, K. L. (2002). Getting more for their dollar: A comparison of the NHS with California's Kaiser Permanente. *British Medical Journal, 324*(7330), 135–141.

Institute for Healthcare Improvement. (2016a). *The IHI triple aim initiative*. Retrieved from http://www.ihi.org/engage/initiatives/tripleaim/Pages/default.aspx

Institute for Healthcare Improvement. (2016b). *Use regular huddles and staff meetings to plan production and to optimize team communication: Improving primary care access*. Retrieved from http://www.ihi.org/resources/Pages/Changes/UseRegularHuddlesandStaffMeetingstoPlanProductionandtoOptimizeTeamCommunication.aspx

Institute for Healthcare Improvement. (2016c). *Optimize the care team: Improving primary care access*. Retrieved from http://www.ihi.org/resources/Pages/Changes/OptimizetheCareTeam.aspx

Institute of Medicine (US). (1999). *To err is human: Building a safer health system*. Washington, DC: National Academies Press.

Institute of Medicine (US). (2001). *Crossing the quality chasm: A new health system for the 21st century*. Washington, DC: National Academies Press.

Institute of Medicine (US). (2006). *Committee on crossing the quality chasm: Adaptation to mental health and addictive disorders. Improving the quality of health care for mental and substance use conditions*. Washington, DC: National Academies Press.

Interprofessional Education Collaborative. (2016). *Core competencies for interprofessional practice: 2016 update*. Washington, DC: Author. Retrieved from https://ipecollaborative.org/uploads/IPEC-2016-Updated-Core-Competencies-Report__final_release_.PDF

Interprofessional Education Collaborative Expert Panel. (2011). *Core competencies for interprofessional practice: Report of an expert panel*. Washington, DC: Interprofessional Education Collaborative. Retrieved from http://www.aacn.nche.edu/education-resources/ipecreport.pdf

Landman, N., Aannestad, L. K., Smoldt, R. K., & Cortese, D. A. (2014). Teamwork in health care. *Nursing Administration Quarterly, 38*(3), 198–205.

Mills, R. J. (2013, November 18). AMA passes recommendations for payment models that support new approaches to team-based health care. *Digital Journal*. Retrieved from http://www.digitaljournal.com/pr/1593833#ixzz2oivWwz3P

Mitchell, P., Wynia, M., Golden, R., McNellis, B., Okun, S., Webb, C. E., et al. (2012). *Core principles & values of effective team-based care*. Washington, DC: Institute of Medicine. Retrieved from https://www.nationalahec.org/pdfs/vsrt-team-based-care-principles-values.pdf

Salas, E., Shuffler, M. L., Thayer, A. L., Bedwell, W. L., & Lazzara, E. H. (2015). Understanding and improving teamwork in organizations: A scientifically based practical guide. *Human Resource Management, 54*(4), 599–622.

Chapter 7
The Business Case for Integrated Behavioral Healthcare Delivery

Ronald O'Donnell

Chapter overview	
	Competencies for calculating program costs, competencies for projecting revenue, competencies for the integrated behavioral health pro forma, and competencies for integrated behavioral health return on investment formula
Key points	*The core competencies for the business case for integrated behavioral healthcare require a synthesis of approaches based on the collaborative care model, the primary care behavioral health model, and value-based behavioral health*
Foundational knowledge and skills	*Ability to design, deliver, and evaluate a business case for integrated behavioral health based on foundational knowledge and skills in calculating program costs, projecting program revenue, completing a business case pro forma, and calculating program return on investment*
Student learning objectives (SLOs)	• *Determine program costs (e.g., staffing productivity), relative value unit, direct, and indirect cost* • *Project program revenue based of fee for service and alternative payment models* • *Complete a program pro forma* • *Complete the steps for return on investment analysis (e.g., plausibility analysis, trend adjustment, event rate and dummy year adjustment, ROI formula)*
Instructional strategies	*Lecture, discussion, digital video media, assigned readings, role play, and presentations*
Evaluating learning	*Quizzes, written assignments, grading discussions, presentations*

R. O'Donnell (✉)
Integrated Behavioral Health Programs, College of Health Solutions, Arizona State University, Phoenix, AZ, USA
e-mail: Ronald.ODonnell@asu.edu

C. R. Macchi, R. Kessler (eds.), *Training to Deliver Integrated Care*,
https://doi.org/10.1007/978-3-319-78850-0_7

Conceptual Shifts That Impact Approaches to Training on the Business Case

The purpose of this chapter is to present training elements used to guide learners on developing effective ways to promote the business case for integrated behavioral healthcare delivery. This chapter defines specific competencies needed for developing and implementing a business case for integrated behavioral health in primary care and identifies related learning objectives, instructional strategies, learning resources, and evaluation techniques. Healthcare systems require financial sustainability – program costs must be covered by organization revenue.

Integrated behavioral health programs can achieve financial sustainability in two ways: (1) generating sufficient revenue to cover the costs of services delivered or (2) demonstrating cost savings based on programs that improve patient health outcomes and result in reduced utilization of high-cost services such as emergency department visits and hospitalizations. Addressing the first approach, Corso, Hunter, Owen, Kallenberg, and Manson (2016) described detailed steps for creating a business case pro forma designed to balance the cost of managing an integrated behavioral health program with revenue for sustainability (Corso et al., 2016). Currently, there is a lack of published research on the use of pro formas to make the business case for integrated behavioral health. The second approach requires a return on investment (ROI) methodology to demonstrate that costs of operating the integrated behavioral health program are offset by cost savings based on reduced utilization and associated costs of care attributed to the program intervention (Lewis, 2012). Over the past 30 years, several studies or reviews have pointed to cost savings associated with behavioral interventions or a medical cost offset that occurs when the cost savings are greater than the cost of the program (Chiles et al., 2002). In spite of these long-standing efforts, a formal business case model for cost-offset or return on investment (ROI) for integrated behavioral health has not been clearly developed and promulgated. In summary, training programs are needed to support the competencies associated with developing a business case for integrated behavioral health using the pro forma and ROI analyses.

Fee-for-Service Versus Value-Based Reimbursement Competencies for integrated behavioral health financial sustainability must also address the movement from fee-for-service (FFS) to value-based healthcare reimbursement. Healthcare payment systems are being redesigned away from FFS payments to value-based payments (Porter & Lee, 2016). Traditional FFS reimbursement is based on retrospective payment for each service based on billing codes that are submitted as a claim to the insurance company (Miller, Ross, Melek, Davis, & Kathol, 2017). This system incentivizes increased volume of services and is in conflict with the Triple Aim (Berwick, Nolan, & Whittington, 2008) goals of improved patient experience of care, population health, and decreased cost of care (Miller et al., 2017). New value-based programs incentivize provider payments based on quality of care (CMS, "What are value-based programs?" (retrieved from https://www.cms.gov/

Medicare/Quality-Initiatives-Patient-Assessment-Instruments/Value-Based-Programs/Value-Based-Programs.html). These programs use alternative payment models (APM) that range from a continuum of modified FFS programs that include FFS and non-FFS payments to global payments in which all reimbursement is based on a predetermined rate based on managing an entire population of patients (Miller et al., 2017). CMS has committed that 90% of Medicare payments will be value-based by 2018, and commercial insurance companies are also moving in this direction (Porter & Lee, 2016). These changes require that leaders must incorporate value-based payment approaches into the business case for integrated behavioral health.

Kathol, deGruy, and Rollman (2014) present guidelines for integrated behavioral health programs transitioning to become a value-based, financially sustainable component of primary care. Value-based payment requires that providers and administrators deliver the highest quality of care with the most efficient resources at the lowest cost (Basu et al., 2017). Kathol et al. (2014) define value-based integrated behavioral health as a population health management model that includes (1) identification and risk stratification of complex, high-cost patients, (2) stepped-care using a team with professional expertise matched to the patient severity/risk stratification, (3) evidence-based behavioral treatments, (4) cross-disciplinary case managers, and (5) clearly defined program outcomes that address both clinical and financial key performance indicators.

Comparing Two Models of Integrated Behavioral Health The business case must also address the model of integrated behavioral health delivery, since the model determines program costs, revenue, and ROI. There are two predominant models of integrated behavioral health: (1) the primary care behavioral health (PCBH) model (Robinson & Reiter, 2016) and the collaborative care model (CoCM) best represented by the AIMS (Advancing Integrated Mental Health Solutions) Center at the University of Washington (https://aims.uw.edu). The PCBH model is based on the inclusion of a behavioral health consultant (BHC[1]) as a member of the primary care team and seeing patients within the primary care clinic office, often via a warm handoff from the primary care physician (PCP) (Robinson & Reiter, 2016). The PCBH serves as a consultant to the primary care team and provides brief, time-limited behavioral treatments to patients. The PBCH BHC is a generalist able to assess and treat a wide range of behavioral conditions, lifestyle behaviors, and medication adherence issues. The CoCM model is also team-based, involving the PCP, a psychiatric consultant, and a behavioral health provider (BHP) more commonly referred to as a care manager (CM). The CoCM incorporated the population health management model recommended by Kathol et al. (2014) as a critical component of value-based care. Consolidated medical record data such as diagnoses, utilization, and cost is used to prospectively identify high-risk patient populations, such as patients diagnosed with diabetes and depression. The CoCM care manager (CM)

[1] Other models of integrated behavioral healthcare refer to the role as a behavioral health provider (BHP). This is the term used in this chapter except when referring to the PCBH model.

develops a plan to address medical and behavioral conditions and follows the patient, usually by phone, using a patient registry to track patient-reported outcomes. The CoCM model also uses a psychiatrist, psychiatric nurse practitioner, or physician assistant to help the patient to manage medication effects and side effects.

Additional features included in the CoCM model make it more difficult to implement than the PCBH model. The CoCM model requires a population health component and related costs such as predictive modeling to identify high-cost patients, a patient registry to track patient outcomes, and the information technology and finance infrastructure necessary for ROI analysis. However, the population health management component of the CoCM model is necessary for achieving cost savings related to decreased utilization (Kathol et al., 2014). The CoCM and related population health management programs have demonstrated significant ROI, whereas the PCBH model has not.

In terms of the revenue-generating component of financial sustainability, CMS has developed three new billing codes that apply to the CoCM model and one new code for the PCBH model (Basu et al., 2017). The PCBH model also may utilize CMS health and behavior codes and/or psychotherapy codes, with significant variation between states and payers in which reimbursement codes are available. Figure 7.1 compares the costs/revenues of the CoCM and PCBH models.

Basu et al. (2017) evaluated the financial impact of behavioral health integration into primary care, comparing the PCBH and CoCM models, using a microsimulation model. The financial modeling was based on extensive cost and revenue assumptions and based on the CMS reimbursement codes designed for the CoCM model. Their results favored the CoCM over the PCBH model with higher projected net revenue; however, the assumptions and design of the microsimulation model, based on the CMS CoCM codes, may not represent the actual financial sustainability of the PCBH model.

Business Case Pro Forma Approach The business case pro forma approach described in Corso et al. (2016) is an excellent resource for determining the financial sustainability of the PCBH model. The business case for the CoCM model is available from the AIMS Center (AIMS Center, building the business case for value-based integrated care, retrieved from https://aims.uw.edu/collaborative-care/building-business-case-cost-effectiveness-studies-collaborative-care). The AIMS Center resources also include a pro forma for the CoCM model, the Financial Modeling Workbook (http://aims.uw.edu/collaborative-care/financing-strategies/financial-modeling-workbook). The AIM Center includes approaches for calculating return on investment based on reduced utilization and related costs of care, as does Lewis (2012).

In conclusion, learners need to appreciate that a successful integrated behavioral health program is much broader than applying a single clinical intervention and needs to include skills in developing the business case for integrated care. The learner must learn to calculate program costs, revenue, and potential cost savings based on the model of integrated behavioral healthcare. In addition, the learner will

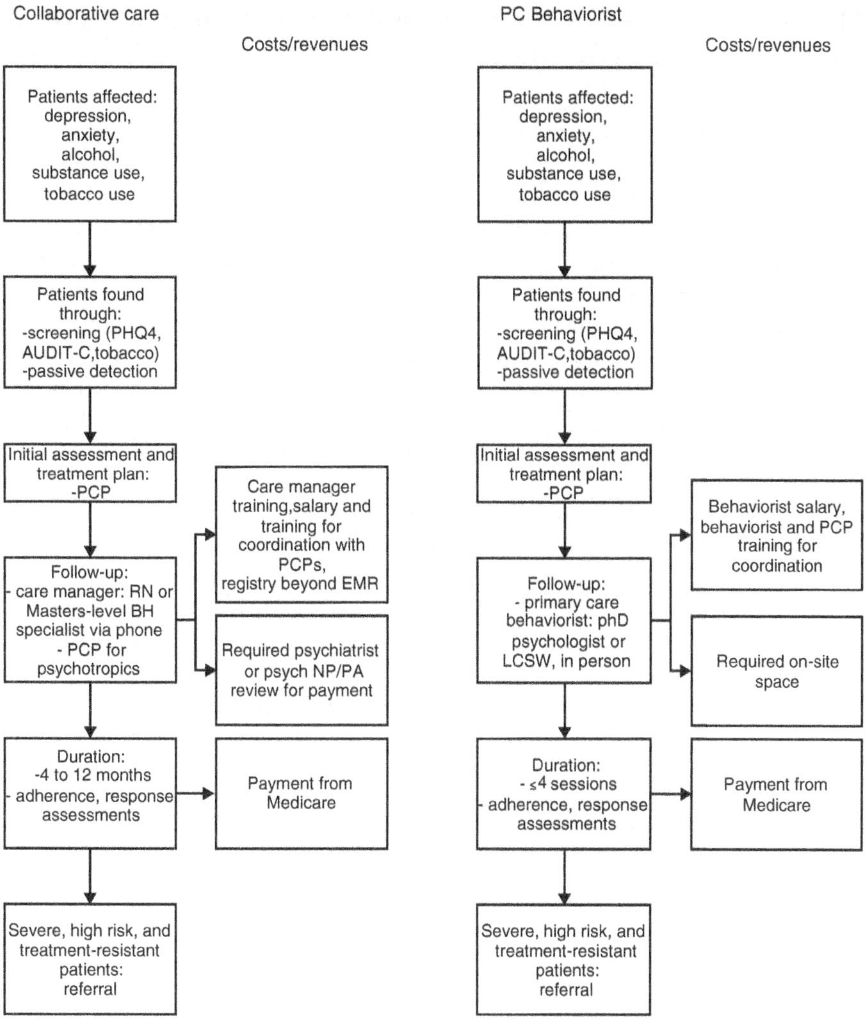

Fig. 7.1 Integrated behavioral health models, costs, and revenues

need to incorporate emerging value-based payment models into their design for the business case for integrated behavioral healthcare. This chapter incorporates elements of both the PCBH and CoCM models of integrated behavioral health. The business case model in this chapter is also based on the Kathol et al. (2014) value-based model for integrated behavioral health. The PCBH and COCM are combined into elements to generate a single business case that calculates the costs to deliver the integrated behavioral health program, the revenue generated by the program, and the cost savings or ROI attributable to the program.

Historical Approaches and Contemporary Movement of Core Competencies for IBH Management

The emphasis on competencies for integrated behavioral health to date has been on clinical competencies for behavioral health providers (Hoge, Morris, Laraia, Pomerantz, & Farley, 2014; McDaniel et al., 2014; Miller et al., 2016). Table 7.1 lists the competencies for clinical providers in primary care based on these authors.

The emphasis of these guidelines is on clinical rather than management competencies. McDaniel et al. (2014) move beyond clinical competencies to address several aspects of management competencies for successful behavioral health integration including: leadership and administration (e.g., organization structure, practice facilitation, strategic planning, organization policy and training), advocacy, and practice management. The practice management competencies include: practice needs assessment, population health management, payment, confidentiality, and technology (McDaniel et al., 2014).

Beacham et al. (2017) proposed competencies for preparing psychologists for leadership in the Patient Centered Medical Home (PCMH). The competency domains are (1) psychological practice in primary care, (2) interprofessional collaborative practice, (3) PCMH guidelines and standards, and (4) psychological practice in primary care. Clearly defined competencies for the *financial management* of integrated behavioral health programs necessary for the design and evaluation of programs are crucial but have not yet been developed.

Practitioner Performance Barriers to Integration

To date, the combined PCBH and COCM have not been widely and systematically integrated in practice, resulting in a lack of models that combine revenue-generating and cost-saving approaches to the business case for integrated behavioral health. A combined model has the potential to incorporate the best components from the PCBH and CoCM models while overcoming each model's limitations. The PCBH model based on a BHC seeing patients who present via a warm handoff is a frequent model in practice and typically does not include a population health management component. The CoCM has proven sustainable in primary care settings and represents the majority of published research on integrated behavioral health (Gerrity, 2016) but has not been broadly implemented in practice. The clinical competencies of both the PCBH model and collaborative care model are well defined (Ratzliff et al., 2016; Robinson & Reiter, 2016), but the management-related competencies for developing the business case for a combined PCBH and CoCM are not yet articulated.

A synthesis of the PCBH and CoCM approaches allows the best components of each model to be integrated into a systematic, organized, and sustainable model of care. The business case for the PCBH model is largely based on revenue from

Table 7.1 Comparison of competencies for clinical providers in primary care

	Assessment	Communication	Teamwork	Care delivery	Interprofessional	Culture
Hoge et al. (2014)	Screening and assessment	Interpersonal communication	Collaboration and teamwork	Intervention	Care planning and collaboration	Cultural competence
Miller et al. (2016)	Identify and assess Engage and activate	Communicate effectively	Work as primary care team member	Provide efficient and effective care	Understand, value, and adapt diverse professional cultures	Provide culturally responsive care
McDaniel et al. (2014)	Application: assessment	Relationships	Relationships teaching and supervision	Science/research and evaluation Application: intervention	Systems relationships: interprofessionalism	Professionalism: cultural diversity

submitting bills and reimbursement for clinical services. The business case for the COCM and value-added model is based on revenue plus the cost savings and ROI as patient health improves and high-cost services, such as emergency department and hospital days, are reduced significantly post-intervention. In addition, CMS has implemented new fee-for-service reimbursement codes specifically designed for the CoCM, further strengthening the business case. This hybrid model represents the new era of value-based business case competencies for integrated behavioral health.

Training and Skill Acquisition

Training and skill acquisition are categorized into four domains: (1) calculating program costs, (2) projecting revenue, (3) completing the pro forma, and (4) calculating cost savings and ROI. Tables 7.2, 7.3, 7.4, and 7.5 identify learning activities and learner assessments for each. The learning activities and assessment techniques are designed for application within in-person (classroom), online, or hybrid (classroom and online) education and training programs. For example, a "discussion" can take place in a live classroom or on a discussion board in an online learning platform. Additional learning activities include:

- Reading publications, guidelines, and research studies on the business case for integrated behavioral health is completed prior to and during training.
- Identifying and studying relevant webpages of organizations that focus on business case development or tools for developing the business case provide learners the ability to return to these sites over time as they practice and refine their skills as new innovations emerge.
- Discussions between the trainer and learners are useful to address key topics and questions raised by the learners.
- Written assignments are focused on the design and analysis of pro forma and ROI calculations.
- Role-play presentations of a completed business case by the learners improve competency to deliver a proposal to key stakeholders in practice.
- Quizzes or exams are useful to demonstrate acquisition of competencies and evaluate both learner progress and training effectiveness.

These teaching strategies are applicable to classroom-based, online, or combined hybrid courses given the availability of both asynchronous (e.g., discussion threads) and synchronous (e.g., live group webinars) technologies in education.

Domain 1: *Competencies for calculating program costs* (Table 7.2) include defining the salary and benefit costs for staffing (BHP/care manager), establishing productivity standards for the PCBH BHC warm handoff and CoCM care manager patient follow-up and outreach activities. Competencies for defining relative value units, costs per unit (direct and indirect), are also included in this domain. The training for these objectives is based on readings and assignments derived from Corso et al. (2016) and from the AIMS Center Financial Modeling Workbook (AIMS

Table 7.2 Domain 1: Competencies for calculating program costs

Competency	Description	Learning objectives	Learning activities	Measurement
BHP, care manager, health coach staffing	BHP salary and benefits	Describe how to evaluate and project BHP, care manager, health coach salary, and benefits based on job description	Search national and local resources to identify salaries for BHP, care manager, etc. Calculate benefits based on organization standards Calculate total cost per FTE Complete summary worksheet	Completed worksheet with sources, salaries, benefits, and total cost Quiz Class role-play presentation Class discussion
BHP productivity	BHP projected patient direct contact hours, consultation, education, etc.	Describe how to develop and manage BHP productivity targets for patient contact hours and other duties (consultation, training, etc.)	Define productivity based on BHP target patient contact hours, types of patient contact (assessment, brief individual or group treatment, consultation, training, documentation, etc.) Complete summary worksheet	Completed BHP productivity worksheet Quiz Class role-play presentation Class discussion
Care manager and/or health coach productivity	Care manager/health coach patient outreach, screening, and patient contact hours (in-person and telephonic) Consultation, documentation, and scheduling	Describe how to estimate care manager/ health coach staffing based on expected number of PHM patients identified, engaged, and continuing in care management follow-up Define care manager consultation, documentation, and other activities	Define productivity based on PHM patient identification, stratification, and projected enrollment Calculate projected patient contacts/services for each phase of PHM (outreach, engagement, enrollment, treatment)	Completed care manager and/or health coach productivity worksheet Quiz Class role-play presentation Class discussion
Relative value unit	RVU is national standard for measuring base unit of clinician work	Describe how to research and calculate RVUs in healthcare	Readings on RVU's Complete RVU calculations for BHP and other positions if applicable	Completed RVU worksheet for each applicable clinician Quiz Class role-play presentation Class discussion
Costs per unit: direct and indirect costs	Direct costs outside of BHP and care manager staffing: supplies, patient screening, patient materials, laptop, CMEs. Consulting with other departments, e.g., IT consulting on patient registry, finance and actuary consulting on predictive modeling for complex patient identification and stratification. Indirect costs include overhead percentage, depreciation	Describe how to identify and quantify direct and indirect program costs	Readings on components of direct and indirect costs Readings of sample direct and indirect costs	Completed summary worksheet of direct and indirect program costs Quiz Class role-play presentation Class discussion

Table 7.3 Domain 2: Competencies for projecting revenue

Competency	Description and Resources	Learning Objectives	Learning Activities	Measurement
Rates and codes for billing	Reimbursement codes by payer, reimbursement code and type, and considerations Rules and regulations for billing	Identify reimbursement codes and associated revenue based on payer, rules, and regulations	General readings on rates and coding for billing Research on local rates and codes for billing	Completed worksheet on billing and coding Quiz Class role-play presentation Class discussion
Maximizing reimbursement through fee schedules and provider type	Fiscal planning based on considerations of provider type and associated fee schedule by payer type	Evaluate provider types and revenue codes to assist in decision-making	Identify rates and coding for billing by type of provider Complete analysis of total costs by type of provider Summary worksheet of comparison provider type and cost	Completed worksheet of provider type and reimbursement based on local billing and coding Quiz Class role-play presentation Class discussion
Alternative payment models and merit based incentive programs	Alternatives to fee-for-service reimbursement such as capitation and merit-based incentive programs	Describe approaches to alternatives payment and merit-based incentive program	Readings on alternative payment and merit-based incentives in general and specific to behavioral health Research websites on alternative payment and merit-based incentive programs	Summary paper describing key components of alternative payment and merit-based incentive programs Quiz Class role-play presentation Class discussion

Table 7.4 Domain 3: Competencies for integrated behavioral health business case pro forma

Competency	Description and resources	Learning objectives	Learning activities	Measurement
Pro forma	Summary document that shows cost and revenue calculations to be used to plan and monitor program finances. Elements include total visit types and reimbursement, BHP and care manager revenue, total net revenue	Demonstrate how to complete a pro forma for an integrated behavioral health program in primary care	Readings on pro forma development Review examples of pro forma Complete pro forma based on worksheets completed on billing rates and reimbursement by provider, total direct and indirect costs	Completed pro forma Quiz Class role-play presentation Class discussion
Program fiscal cost savings and ROI	Formulas (annual and monthly): gain from program minus the cost of program divided by the cost of program	Demonstrate how to calculate fiscal cost savings and ROI	Readings on how to calculate annual cost of program and annual revenue Readings on how to complete summary ROI formula for program	Completed program fiscal cost savings and ROI summary worksheet Quiz Class role-play presentation Class discussion

Table 7.5 Domain 4: Competencies for integrated behavioral health return on investment formula

Competency	Description and resources	Learning objectives	Learning activities	Measurement
Plausibility testing: the event rate and the dummy year adjustment	Plausibility testing is a methodology to construct a ROI model consistent with the expected impact of an intervention on utilization pre- versus post-intervention Event rate and dummy year adjustment are methods to accurately determine cases to include in the ROI analysis	Describe the rationale and key components of plausibility testing Describe how the event rate and dummy year Adjustment will be used to adjust for utilization and cost pre- and post-intervention in the ROI analysis	Readings on plausibility testing, event rate, and dummy year adjustment Complete worksheet based on fictional pre- and post-utilization and cost data	Completed worksheet on plausibility testing and dummy year adjustment Class role-play presentation and discussion/feedback Quiz
Seven rules of plausibility and case studies	The seven rules of plausibility are often violated (case studies will be reviewed) Approaches to applying the seven rules successfully will be evaluated	Describe the seven rules of plausibility and case studies that demonstrate violation of one or more of the rules and case studies that meet all seven rules	Readings on the seven rules of plausibility. Read case studies that reflect violations of one or more of the rules and that reflect meeting all rules	Class discussion and feedback Quiz
Utilization trend adjustment	Methods of adjusting utilization based on trends that influence utilization such as annual inflation, changes in insurance benefit, and outlier cases	Describe methods of evaluating and adjusting utilization trend Describe methods of adjusting projected trend for ROI formula based on evaluation	Readings on utilization trend adjustment Complete worksheets based on fictional data to adjust for trend in data	Class discussion and feedback Completed worksheets on utilization trend adjustment Quiz
ROI formula	The formula for ROI is the cost savings attributable to the intervention (defined as post-utilization cost minus the pre-utilization cost divided by the total cost of the program)	Describe the formula for ROI Complete a ROI formula based on a case study simulation	Readings on ROI formula calculation Complete worksheets for ROI formula based on fictional data	Completed worksheet Class discussion and feedback Quiz

Center, 2017 retrieved from http://aims.uw.edu/collaborative-care/financing-strategies/financial-modeling-workbook). The readings provide the basis for learning about the key components of a pro forma for the business case. Learners are required to develop and complete worksheets for BHP costs and productivity (e.g., pro forma, return on investment (ROI), cost savings, and cost offset) (Corso et al., 2016) that are used for a final pro forma based on fictional raw data. Class role-play activities (tailored to classroom or online learning) are included based on a simulation of a primary care stakeholder meeting in which students present their pro forma to peers and/or the instructor for discussion and feedback. These discussion sessions simulate questions and feedback that are critical to designing a business case in integrated care. Written exercises/grading rubrics and quizzes are included as an additional assessment of content knowledge.

Domain 2: Competencies for projecting revenue (Table 7.3) include identifying billing codes for reimbursement rates and maximizing reimbursement through fee schedules and provider types, and alternative payment models are critical for income to support the business case. Learning activities include readings and assignments derived from Corso et al. (2016) complimented with examples from other organizations such as the AIMS Center (AIMS Center, 2016 retrieved from https://aims.uw.edu) and SAMHSA (SAMHSA, 2016 retrieved from http://www.integration.samhsa.gov/financing). The learning activities include readings combined with focused and detailed review of reimbursement information from agencies that are local to the learner practice settings. Billing and reimbursement procedures and codes and eligible provider types can vary significantly between states and require learning activities customized to the clinic state. Learning activities include completing worksheets based on case studies with adjustments for each specific state. Reading assignments are complimented by directed searches of organization websites with detailed billing information for each state. This learning objective is a necessary step before completing the next Domain 3 – competencies for the pro forma – as projected revenue data are used to complete the pro forma.

Domain 3: Competencies for integrated behavioral health business case pro forma (Table 7.4) learning activities include readings and assignments derived from Corso et al. (2016) complimented with examples from other organizations such as the AIMS Center (AIMS Center, 2016 retrieved from https://aims.uw.edu) and SAMHSA (SAMHSA, 2016 retrieved from http://www.integration.samhsa.gov/financing). Students complete worksheets for a pro forma based on fictional data and then present the pro forma in a role-play, engage in discussion, and receive feedback. A quiz is also administered to evaluate this activity. The pro forma is a critical component of finalizing cost and revenue for the integrated behavioral health model.

Domain 4: Competencies for integrated behavioral health return on investment formula (Table 7.5) are comprised of the concept of plausibility testing, including the event rate and dummy year adjustment, seven rules of plausibility, utilization trend adjustment, and ROI formula. The learning activities include completing worksheets for each of these components based on fictional data from a case study. Learning activities also include discussion and feedback, role-play presentation of the final ROI formula, and a quiz.

Measurement: Evaluation

The learning activities are evaluated by a combination of measurements to evaluate competencies. The measurement approach is based on developing measureable assessments for each key learning activity. The types of assessment include grading of worksheets or papers, class discussion and feedback (in-person discussion or online via discussion board), and role-play exercises (in-person live presentations or online via group synchronous or asynchronous presentations and feedback) and quizzes. This criterion-based approach to measurement and evaluation is critical in demonstrating competencies in writing exercises, discussion, and feedback, and webinar role-play presentations and feedback reflect the need to demonstrate competencies across these common scenarios.

Examples of measurement and evaluation are included in Appendices A, B, and C from the Arizona State University Integrated Behavioral Health program. Appendix A is a discussion board grading rubric. This rubric covers quality, clarity and mechanics, references and support, and follow-up for an online discussion. Appendix B includes assignment instructions and a grading rubric for a written assignment "Integrated Behavioral Health Intervention Utilization, Cost, Cost Savings and Return on Investment Results, and Analysis" from a course titled "Cost Offset and Return on Investment." Appendix C provides a sample quiz question from the same course. Appendix D is a group activity assignment on the topic: Billing and Reimbursement in Integrated Healthcare, from a course titled "Behavioral Health Management." In this assignment students are assigned to groups and meet on a webcam platform to present and discuss their proposal for the upcoming written assignment.

These examples in Tables A through D are based on an online learning approach but can be easily modified to an in-person training or education approach. These examples were selected to demonstrate measurement and evaluation of strategic approaches to teaching based on completing written assignments, discussions, group activity, and quiz. For example, online continuing education programs are often asynchronous and do not have the capacity for instructor grading of written assignments. In this case the written assignments can be readily adapted to an online continuing education program by using online quizzes with applied questions in formats such as true or false, multiple choice, matching, and fill in the blank in order to test the competency for each component of the written assignment. The group activities can be adopted for online continuing education programs that do not have the capacity for synchronous group meetings by using simulation exercises. These may be constructed in written form such as case studies, in digital video form with recorded group activity vignettes, and by virtual reality programs that present interpersonal scenarios. In each of these examples, the grading rubrics can be readily adapted to online synchronous, asynchronous, or in-person training using principles of effective grading rubrics (Van Leusen, 2013 retrieved from https://teachonline.asu.edu/2013/08/assessments-with-rubrics/#more-2246).

For in-person training programs, the written assignments can be readily adapted for participants to complete written exercises of components alone or in small groups. The group activity exercise is ideal for in-person training and affords the opportunity for students to both demonstrate content mastery and to practice many professional activities (e.g., completing a pro forma based on existing data and then role-play presentations of the completed pro forma to peer trainees). Assessing competencies may occur through trainer observations and rubric ratings for in-person group activity and through peer ratings. Similarly, discussing board assignments may be adapted for in-person training programs by having trainees conduct live discussions that trainers or peer trainees observe and rate using rubrics. Trainers may use peer trainee ratings for large groups of trainees. The trainer can ask each group to have the leader provide a brief, structured summary to the entire group of trainees that the trainer can evaluate for each group. Creative use of mobile phone or tablet apps during training that are designed for trainees to enter responses to questions related to target competencies create a written record for grading competencies.

Summary This model for training the value-based business case for integrated behavioral health combines the strengths of the PCBH and COCM within the framework of value-based, population health management approaches proposed by Kathol et al. (2014). The PCBH is necessary for active patient management using PCP-led, team-based care in the PCMH. In addition, the PCBH BHC is ideally suited to provide consultation, training, and education to the PCMH team on all aspects of integrated behavioral care. The CoCM care manager is necessary to deliver the patient outreach and long-term follow-up treatment essential to achieving improved health, decreased utilization, and resultant cost savings.

Appendix A: Degree Program Discussion Board Rubric

Criteria	Unacceptable	Acceptable	Good	Excellent
Quality of initial post (2 points)	Post meets one or fewer of the four criteria or did not submit (0 points)	Post meets two of the four criteria (1 point)	Post meets three of the four criteria (1.5 points)	Initial post meets all of the following criteria • Is well developed • Fully addresses all aspects of the discussion board question • Meets criteria for substantive (**salutations and references do not count toward minimum word requirements**) • Post is factually correct (2 points)
References and support (.5 points)	Post incorporates zero course materials or did not submit (0 points)	Post incorporates one piece of information or meets one of the three required criteria (0.1 point)	Post incorporates two pieces of information or meets two of the three required criteria (0.3 point)	Post incorporates three pieces of information from course materials (e.g. assigned readings, lectures, etc.) and meets all of the following criteria: • Includes in-text citations • Includes reference list • At least one reference is from an assigned reading (0.5 point)
Clarity and mechanics	Post meets two or fewer of the required criteria or did not submit (0 points)	Post meets three of the five required criteria (0.1 point)	Post meets four of the five required criteria (0.3 point)	Post meets all of the following criteria: • Reference is in APA style (indentation not required due to formatting limitation of discussion board) • In-text citation is in APA style • Has no more than two errors in clarity/mechanics and/or grammatical/spelling errors • Communicates in a friendly and courteous manner • Post is well organized and easy to read (0.5 point)

Follow-up postings	Post meets two or fewer of the required criteria or post does not add to the discussion or did not submit (0 points)	Response post adds to the discussion and post meets three to four of the nine required criteria (0.5 point)	Response post adds to the discussion and post meets five to six of the nine required criteria (0.75 point)	Response post adds to the discussion through the provision of a new idea or concept based on course content and meets six of the nine following criteria: • Is well developed • Meets criteria for substantive (**salutations and references do not count toward minimum word requirements**) • Post is factually correct • Post does not merely restate the student's initial post • Includes in-text citations and/or a reference list • Reference list and/or in-text citations are in APA style • Post is free of grammatical/spelling errors • Communicates in a friendly and courteous manner • Post is well organized and easy to read (1 point)

Appendix B: Assignment Instructions and Grading Rubric for Written Assignment: Integrated Behavioral Health Intervention Utilization, Cost, Cost Savings, and Return on Investment Results and Analysis (25 points)

Assignment #1 Instructions

Complete a proposal for the design, implementation, and evaluation of an *integrated behavioral health intervention* designed to result in cost savings and a return on investment. The intervention must address at least two conditions: one must be medical (e.g., diabetes, hypertension) and one must be behavioral (e.g., depression, anxiety, substance use disorder). The intervention should be based on the population health management (PHM) model. Examples and instructions for the PHM model are included in the assigned readings. You will write the proposal as an integrated behavioral health provider. The intended audience for this report is the CEO for a Patient-Centered Medical Home and Accountable Care Organization primary care clinic network. The proposal must include each of the following sections:

Program/Intervention Costs List staffing, administrative support, supplies, physician and nurse time, data entry and analysis, etc. You must use dollar estimates for each cost category and a grand total for program costs.

Pre-intervention (Baseline) Utilization and Cost List each category of utilization and associated dollar cost (e.g., physician visits, emergency department visits, hospital admissions and days, pharmacy, specialist referral visits, labs, and imaging). Include aggregate mean utilization and cost for at least 2 years and ideally 3 years pre-intervention. For each unit of service, assign a specific dollar amount. Compute the total pre-intervention cost based on the mean (average) annual utilization multiplied by the unit cost for each category.

Post-Intervention Utilization and Cost List each category of utilization and associated dollar cost (e.g., physician visits, emergency department visits, hospital admissions and days, pharmacy, specialist referral visits, labs, and imaging). Include aggregate mean utilization and cost for at least 1 year post-intervention. For each unit of service, assign a specific dollar amount. Compute the total post-intervention cost based on the mean (average) annual utilization multiplied by the unit cost for each category.

Return on Investment Calculation Use the formula listed in the readings to calculate return on investment: total cost savings (pre-intervention costs minus post-intervention costs) divided by the total cost of the intervention.

ROI Analysis Executive summary: brief summary of entire project, rationale for leadership investment in project, overall benefits, and long-term sustainability of program.

Assignment #1 Grading Rubric (Edited, Selected Sections Only for Illustrative Purposes)

Item	**Excellent 2.0**	**Fair 1.0**	**Unacceptable 0**
Problem statement	Clear statement of need based on evidence for high costs for the selected conditions and population	Vague or partial statement of need based on evidence for high costs for the selected conditions and population	No statement of need based on evidence for high costs for the selected conditions and population
Population	All key elements described: age, gender, ethnicity, setting	Partial description of key elements: age, gender, ethnicity, setting	No description of key elements: age, gender, ethnicity, setting
Patient identification	Clear description of how patients will be identified based on more than one criteria, such as patient self-report measures, claims data, lab, or diagnostic data in the electronic medical record, physician referral	Vague or partial description of how patients will be identified based on more than one criteria, such as patient self-report measures, claims data, lab, or diagnostic data in the electronic medical record, physician referral	No description of how patients will be identified based on more than one criteria, such as patient self-report measures, claims data, lab, or diagnostic data in the electronic medical record, physician referral
	Excellent 5.0	**Fair 4.0**	**Poor 3.0**
Program costs	Clear description of costs for program including staffing, administrative support, supplies, physician and nurse time, data entry and analysis, etc. Use dollar estimates for each cost category and a grand total for program costs	Vague or partial description of costs for program including staffing, administrative support, supplies, physician and nurse time, data entry and analysis, etc. Incomplete use of dollar estimates for each cost category and a grand total for program costs	Poor description of costs for program including staffing, administrative support, supplies, physician and nurse time, data entry and analysis, etc. No use of dollar estimates for each cost category and a grand total for program costs

(continued)

Item	Excellent 2.0	Fair 1.0	Unacceptable 0
Pre- and post-intervention utilization and cost intervention costs)	Clear, detailed description of each key type of utilization such as physician visits, emergency department visits, hospital admissions and days, pharmacy, specialist referral visits, labs, and imaging that you will report based on the mean number of visits per patient for at least 1 year prior to the intervention and 1 year post-intervention. For each unit of service, assign a specific dollar amount, and compute the total cost of pre- and post-intervention based on utilization. Includes a total dollar amount for pre-intervention utilization/costs and post-intervention utilization/costs	Vague or partial description of each key type of utilization such as physician visits, emergency department visits, hospital admissions and days, pharmacy, specialist referral visits, labs, and imaging that you will report based on the mean number of visits per patient for at least 1 year prior to the intervention and 1 year post-intervention. Unclear description of how each unit of service is assigned a specific dollar amount and unclear computation of the total cost of pre- and post-intervention based on utilization. Unclear plan to have a total dollar amount for pre-intervention utilization/costs and post-intervention utilization/costs	Poor description of each key type of utilization such as physician visits, emergency department visits, hospital admissions and days, pharmacy, specialist referral visits, labs, and imaging that you will report based on the mean number of visits per patient for at least 1 year prior to the intervention and 1 year post-intervention. Poor description of how each unit of service you will assign a specific dollar amount and compute the total cost of pre- and post-intervention based on utilization. Lacking plan to have a total dollar amount for pre-intervention utilization/costs and post-intervention utilization/costs
ROI calculation	Clear description of the ROI calculation based on the formula listed in the readings to calculate return on investment: total cost savings (pre-intervention costs minus post-intervention costs) divided by the total cost of the intervention	Vague or partial description of the ROI based on the formula listed in the readings to calculate return on investment: total cost savings (pre-intervention costs minus post-intervention costs) divided by the total cost of the intervention	No description of ROI based on the formula listed in the readings to calculate return on investment: total cost savings (pre-intervention costs minus post-intervention costs) divided by the total cost of the intervention

Appendix C: Sample Quiz Question

Multiple choice: PCMH and diabetes cost savings
Points:**1**

Question	In the article by Wang et. al., "Patient-centered medical home impact on health plan members with diabetes," Table 3, which of the following outcome measures was not associated with a significant reduction in costs between baseline and at least one year 1, 2, or 3 in the study for the PCMH?
Answer	Total medical care PMPM Inpatient PMPM ED PMPM ✔ Pharmacy (Rx) PMPM

Appendix D: Group Activity: Billing and Reimbursement in Integrated Healthcare (Edited)

Overview

In this assignment, you will research billing codes and reimbursement for integrated healthcare services in a primary care clinic. This group activity is designed to help you prepare for written assignment #1.

Instructions

In this week Chap. 7 in Corso et al. (2016) "Integrating Behavioral Health into the Medical Home," a strong emphasis is on analyzing reimbursement rates as a component of your business case or integrated behavioral health. In this group assignment, I would like each of you to research the billing codes specific to the institution, payer, and provider license for either (a) your current clinical practice (if you work in a clinical setting) or (b) a primary care Accountable Care Organization (ACO) clinic in your state (for students who do not work in a clinic). Approach this with the assumption that you are the clinic leader interested in developing/enhancing integrated behavioral health in your clinic. You plan to evaluate which reimbursement codes your clinic is eligible for and what types of clinicians are eligible for reimbursement for reimbursement codes that are available in your clinic.

Evaluate each of the specific codes listed below for your clinic scenario. Which codes are eligible for reimbursement? For those codes that your clinic is eligible for, answer these questions: What provider license types? What payers? What reimbursement rates (if available)?

Health and Behavior Codes
Psychotherapy Codes
Screening, Brief Assessment, Referral and Treatment Codes
Wellness Codes
Screening and Prevention Codes
Care Coordination/Chronic Care Management

The presentation should be brief, simple, and delivered as if you were in a team meeting in a clinic setting making your presentation to your integrated behavioral health "team." You are making a presentation to your "team" based on your initial analysis and expect questions, discussion, and next steps.

Instructions for Discussion Board Post and Substantive Reply

After the meeting is completed, each student should write a summary post on the group discussion board that describes his/her experience in the group. Was the group meeting helpful? Were there challenges? Describe how the group discussion helped to refine your approach to this assignment. Finally, post a brief (one paragraph) summary of your research on reimbursement for services in support of integrated behavioral health in your scenario. What services in support of integrated care are reimbursable in your scenario? Which one's are not?

References

Basu, S., Landon, B., William, J., Bitton, A., Song, Z., & Phillips, R. (2017). Behavioral health integration into primary care: A microsimulation of financial implications for practices. *Journal of General Internal Medicine*, published online doi: https://doi.org/10.1007/s11606-017-4177-0j.

Beacham, A., Khatri, P., Reimer, D., Sickle, K., Ali, M., Farber, E., et al. (2017). Meeting evolving workforce needs: Preparing psychologists for leadership in the patient-centered medical home. *American Psychologist, 72*(1), 42–54.

Berwick, D., Nolan, T., & Whittington, J. (2008). The triple aim: Care, health and cost. *Health Affairs, 27*(3), 759–769. https://doi.org/10.1377/hlthaff.27.3.759.

Chiles, J. A., Lambert, M. J., & Hatch, L. (2002). Medical costs offset: a review of the impact of psychological interventions on medical utilization over the past three decades. In N. A. Cummings, W. T. O'Donohue, & K. E. Ferguson (Eds.), *The impact of medical cost offset on practice and research: making it work for you* (pp. 47–56). Reno: Context Press.

Corso, K., Hunter, C., Owen, D., Kallenberg, G., & Manson, L. (2016). *Integrating behavioral health into the medical home: A rapid implementation guide*. Williamsport, PA: Greenbranch.

Gerrity, M. (2016). *Evolving models of behavioral health integration: Evidence update 2010–2015*. Rockport, MD: Milbank Memorial Fund.

Hoge, M., Morris, J., Laraia, M., Pomerantz, A., & Farley, T. (2014). *Core competencies for integrated behavioral health and primary care*. Washington, DC: SAMHSA-HRSA Center for Integrated Health Solutions.

Kathol, R. G., deGruy, F., & Rollman, B. L. (2014). Value-based financially sustainable behavioral health components in patient-centered medical homes. *The Annals of Family Medicine, 12*(2), 172–175. https://doi.org/10.1370/afm.1619.

Lewis, A. (2012). *Why nobody believes the numbers: Distinguishing fact from fiction in population health management*. New Jersey: Wiley.

McDaniel, S., Grus, C., Cubic, B., Hunter, C., Kearney, L., Schuman, C., et al. (2014). Competencies for psychology practice in primary care. *American Psychologist, 69*(4), 409–429.

Miller, B., Gilchrist, E., Ross, K., Wong, S., Blount, A., & Peek, C. (2016). *Core competencies for behavioral health providers working in primary care*. Prepared from the Colorado Consensus Conference.

Miller, B., Ross, K., Melek, S., Davis, M., & Kathol, R. (2017). Payment reform in the Patient-Centered Medical Home: Enabling and sustaining integrated behavioral health care. *American Psychologist, 72*(1), 55–68.

Porter, M., & Lee, T. (2016). From volume to value in health care: The work begins. *JAMA, 316*(1), 1047–1048.

Ratzliff, A., Unutzer, J., Katon, W., & Stephens, K. (2016). *Integrated care: Creating effective mental and primary health care teams* (p. 2016). Hoboken: Wiley.

Robinson, P., & Reiter, J. (2016). *Behavioral consultation and primary care: A guide to integrating services* (2nd ed.). New York: Springer.

Van Leusen, P. (2013). *Assessments with rubrics*. Arizona State University. Teach Online: Resources for Teaching Online. Accessed 25 July 2016 at https://teachonline.asu.edu/2013/08/assessments-with-rubrics/#more-2246.

Chapter 8
Business Entrepreneurship: The Integrated Behavioral Health Business Plan

Ronald O'Donnell and Sue Dahl-Popolizio

Chapter overview	
Domains	*Competencies for a behavioral health business plan, entrepreneurial thinking, and marketing integrated behavioral health programs*
Key points	*The core competencies in entrepreneurship skills for the behavioral healthcare clinician. The course focuses on entrepreneurial skills designed to prepare the behavioral clinician to start a new business venture or revitalize an existing organization or business to meet the needs of the evolving healthcare system and marketplace*
Foundational knowledge and skills	*Ability to design, deliver, and evaluate a realistic business plan that addresses an entrepreneurial opportunity in an integrated healthcare setting. Identify opportunities for business ventures related to gaps in current healthcare services, as well as how to evaluate and revitalize existing businesses or business concepts through process improvement. Present business plan ideas verbally in a PowerPoint pitch, providing hands-on experience in how to convincingly convey their business plan idea.*
Student learning objectives (SLOs)	*Evaluate and explain the range of entrepreneurial opportunities open to behavioral health clinicians Develop a specific entrepreneurial concept based on this evaluation of entrepreneurial opportunities Develop steps and identify resources needed for a start-up business. Create a formal business plan for an integrated medical and behavioral healthcare program. Create strategies to demonstrate the value of a behavioral health clinician in a medical setting with strategies to promote clinical identity in the medical setting. Compose a plan to speak with upper management in healthcare regarding the behavioral care provider's skillset and ability to provide process improvements to their business*
Instructional strategies	*Lecture, discussion, digital video media, assigned readings, role-play, and presentations*
Evaluating learning	*Quizzes, written assignments, grading discussions, presentations*

R. O'Donnell (✉) · S. Dahl-Popolizio
Integrated Behavioral Health Programs, College of Health Solutions,
Arizona State University, Phoenix, AZ, USA
e-mail: Ronald.ODonnell@asu.edu; Sue.Dahlpopolizio@asu.edu

C. R. Macchi, R. Kessler (eds.), *Training to Deliver Integrated Care*,
https://doi.org/10.1007/978-3-319-78850-0_8

Overview

The purpose of this chapter is to present components to be used for trainees to learn how to apply strategies and techniques of business entrepreneurship to integrated behavioral healthcare delivery. This curriculum is an introduction to the essential entrepreneurship skills for the behavioral healthcare clinician or manager. The course focuses on entrepreneurial skills designed to prepare the behavioral clinician to start a new business venture or revitalize an existing organization or business to meet the needs of the evolving healthcare system and marketplace.

The course will present an overview of entrepreneurship as it relates to integrated medical and behavioral health. The course places a major emphasis on the design and development of an integrated behavioral health business plan. The student will have the opportunity to learn how to identify opportunities for business ventures related to gaps in current healthcare services, as well as how to evaluate and revitalize existing businesses or business concepts through strategic business planning. Students present their business plan ideas verbally in a PowerPoint pitch, providing hands-on experience in both written and verbal presentation skills.

Historical Approaches to Education and Training the Integrated Behavioral Health Entrepreneur

Boore and Porter (2011) describe education for entrepreneurship in nursing. They note that the field of social entrepreneurship, the use of entrepreneurial skills to meet social needs or lead transformation of healthcare systems (CCSE, 2001), is applicable to healthcare. They also note that intrapreneurship, when an organization encourages and develops entrepreneurship within the organization staff (NICENT, 2004), is consistent with efforts to innovate in the business of healthcare. Boone and Porter (2011) proposed a comprehensive model of entrepreneurship nursing education that includes learning outcomes, curriculum descriptions, and assessment approaches for entrepreneurship learning outcomes (see Tables 8.1 and 8.2). This appears to be one of the few published curricula for entrepreneurship in healthcare.

Key Conceptual and Operational Shifts in Behavioral Entrepreneurship

Shatz et al. (2014) identifies four solutions designed to address this gap between education and entrepreneurship:

1. Technology transfer offices in universities and companies designed to identify research with commercial potential
2. Entrepreneurship centers in universities to assist academics develop business plans

Table 8.1 Grading rubric for the behavioral health business plan written assignment

Competency	Excellent	Good	Poor
Industry analysis and trends (1–2 pages, 3 points)	Points: 3 (12%) At least eight of ten components included: 1. Your business and industry 2. Your economic sector 3. Your industry 4. Size and growth rate of your industry 5. Sensitivity to economic cycles: your business and industry 6. Technological change 7. Regulation/ certification 8. Supply and distributions channels 9. Financial characteristics 10. Global industry concerns clearly evaluates the standards, trends, and features of your industry. Excellent writing organization, conciseness, and clarity	Points: 2 (8%) At least six of ten components included. Good evaluation of the standards, trends, and features of your industry. Good writing organization, conciseness, and clarity	Points: 1 (4%) Less than six components included. Does not clearly evaluate the standards, trends, and features of your industry. Poor writing organization, conciseness, and clarity
Strategic position and risk assessment (2 pages, 3 points)	Points: 3 (12%) At least five of seven components included: 1. Why should customers buy from you 2. A strategic position defines what you do 3. A strategic position also defines what you don't do 4. Strategic position is more than advertising 5. What kinds of strategic position are here 6. Risks. 7. Balancing risks and opportunities clearly defines your strategic position enables you to clearly and completely know what business you are in. Makes clear that there is no one "correct" strategy, and your strategic position will evolve over time. Excellent assessment of your risks to better reduce potential threats to your success. Excellent writing organization, conciseness, and clarity	Points: 2 (8%) At least four of seven components included. Good defines of your strategic position enables you to know what business you are in. Makes clear that your strategic position will evolve over time. Good assessment of your risks to better reduce potential threats to your success. Good writing organization, conciseness, and clarity	Points: 1 (4%) Less than four components included. Does not clearly define your strategic position or enables you to clearly and completely know what business you are in. Does not make clear that there is no one "correct" strategy, and your strategic position will evolve over time. Poor assessment of your risks to better reduce potential threats to your success. Poor writing organization, conciseness, and clarity
Format and references (2 points)• APA 6th Ed. format• >75% references are <5 years old	Points: 2 (8%) Font, spacing, and APA format, references are correctly formatted with <3 errors	Points: 1 (4%) Font and spacing, font and APA format, references have between three and six errors	Points: 0 (0%) Font, spacing, or APA format, references have more than six errors

Table 8.2 Grading rubric for the behavioral health business plan pitch presentation

Item	Excellent	Good	Fair	Poor
Content design	Points: 4 (20%) Excellent visual design (clearly used tips in Garr Reynolds). Slides are not unnecessarily complicated or "busy" with plenty of white space. Bullets and texts are limited. Excellent use of graphics (numbers, charts, digital images) to convey key points of each slide. Excellent use of consistent color scheme	Points: 3 (15%) Very good visual design (some use of tips in Garr Reynolds). Slides are generally not unnecessarily complicated or "busy" with fair amount of white space. Bullets and texts are limited. Very good use of graphics (numbers, charts, digital images) to convey key points of each slide. Good use of consistent color scheme on majority of slide set	Points: 2 (10%) Fair visual design (did not consistently use tips in Garr Reynolds). Slides are unnecessarily complicated or "busy" with lack of white space. Bullets and texts are used often. Lacking sufficient use of graphics (numbers, charts, digital images) to convey key points of each slide. Inconsistent use of consistent color scheme	Points: 1 (5%) Poor visual design (did not use tips in Garr Reynolds). Slides are very complicated or "busy" with very little white space. Bullets and texts are overused. Poor or no use of graphics (numbers, charts, digital images) to convey key points of each slide. Poor use of consistent color scheme with changes from slide to slide
Delivery presentation	Points: 4 (20%) Excellent demonstration of passion for topic with confidence and enthusiasm evident in verbal presentation. Does not make false or exaggerated claims. Strong start with highly engaging introduction (consider using a story per Garr Reynolds). Clear evidence of practice with slides as evidenced by smooth verbal delivery, excellent transitions between slides	Points: 3 (15%) Good demonstration of passion for topic with some confidence and enthusiasm evident in verbal presentation. Generally, does not make false or exaggerated claims. Good start with engaging introduction (consider using a story per Garr Reynolds). Evidence of practice with slides as evidenced by smooth verbal delivery, generally good transitions between slides	Points: 2 (10%) Generally lacking good passion for topic, some lack of confidence and enthusiasm evident in verbal presentation, and/or some false or exaggerated claims, and/or start is not highly engaging, and/or lack of evidence of practice with slides as evidenced by some discontinuity in verbal delivery, some lack of continuity in transitions between slides	Points: 1 (5%) Generally lacking good passion for topic, some lack of confidence and enthusiasm evident in verbal presentation, and/or some false or exaggerated claims, and/or start is not highly engaging, and/or lack of evidence of practice with slides as evidenced by some discontinuity in verbal delivery, and/or clear lack of continuity in transitions between slides

3. Specialized entrepreneurship programs that provide business education to health care professionals, such as the Duke University Healthcare Innovation and Entrepreneurship course (https://www.coursera.org/learn/healthcare-innovation)
4. Dual degree programs that combine a master degree in healthcare business with a medical degree

Shatz et al. (2014) notes that all of these approaches have limitations in reaching a small audience often restricted to the local university academics, and they are not widely available to practicing physicians and psychologists tasked with design and implementation of health programs. He proposed a solution by developing venture capital (VC) panels in healthcare conferences (Shatz et al. 2014). He identified seven key competencies: (1) define the product or service you are developing, (2) determine market forces and target audience, (3) describe your competitive advantage, (4) the business plan, (5) current and future resources and capabilities, (6) legal consultation, and (7) the art of making a business pitch (Shatz et al. 2014). He notes that even this solution is partial, with impact limited to those interested in venture capital, as opposed to those who implement program within existing organizations.

Practitioner Performance Barriers to Behavioral Entrepreneurship Historically, education and training programs for entrepreneurship in healthcare overall and specifically in behavioral health have been lacking. Shatz et al. (2014) notes a gap between academia and business, with professional healthcare education offering few programs for training healthcare professionals in entrepreneurship. In particular, physicians, psychologists, and other professionals design and implement healthcare programs without adequate business knowledge (Shatz et al. 2014). An article by Cohn and Schwartz (2002) reported that many physicians are not aware of the importance of having a proper business plan for their practice, unable to design one, and subsequently facing financial struggles trying to manage their practice. While there are many business-oriented courses and books on entrepreneurship, there are scant resources for entrepreneurship in healthcare.

The Integrated Behavioral Entrepreneur Business Plan Core Competencies

The core competencies of entrepreneurship include completing a business plan, strategic planning and execution of entrepreneurial activities, and marketing. This section will cover each of these topics in detail, including sample assignment and grading rubrics. This chapter is based on the business plan strategy of Abrams (2014) adapted for the integrated behavioral healthcare industry. The business plan core competencies are relevant to any new proposal by a behavioral health consultant, whether it is within an existing organization or as a consultant or business start-up. This chapter will utilize the sections of a successful business plan described by Abrams (2014) with relevant examples specific to the current and evolving integrated behavioral health marketplace. The chapter will address the steps necessary for an effective business plan by a behavioral health consultant, along with examples of specific strategies and techniques.

The business plan core competencies are based on the components of a business plan (Abrams, 2014):

- Executive summary
- Company description
- Industry trends and analysis
- Target market
- The competition
- Strategic position and risk assessment
- Marketing plan and sales strategy
- Operations
- Technology plan
- Management and organization
- Social responsibility and sustainability
- Development, milestones, and exit plan
- The financials

Executive Summary This is the single most important part of your business plan. Write the executive summary last, after you have carefully completed all other components of the business plan. The executive summary must demonstrate to the reader that:

- Your basic business concept makes sense.
- The business model has been thoroughly planned.
- The management team is capable.
- A clear-cut market exists.
- The business includes competitive advantages.
- Financial projections are realistic.
- The organization has an opportunity to make a financial profit and/or achieve other strategic goals.

The executive summary must be targeted to the intended audience, such as medical director, CEO, CFO, board of directors, or investors. There are two styles of writing a business plan, the synopsis or the narrative summary. The synopsis is a set of conclusions based on each component of the business plan. The narrative summary tells a story with greater passion and engagement. The synopsis is relatively easy to write but may be boring; the narrative requires advanced writing skills and time but may have more impact.

Company Description This section includes the basic details of your business, including what it does and what you have accomplished to date. It includes a **mission statement** that concisely documents the focus and objectives of your company. The description should include:

- Company name
- Company's objectives/mission statement
- Legal issues
- Products and services
- Management/leadership
- Business location
- Development stage and milestones achieved to date
- Financial status

Industry Analysis and Trends This section evaluates the standards, trends, and features of integrated behavioral health in the healthcare industry. This section should capitalize on trends in healthcare that are drivers for integrated behavioral health, such as the rise of chronic disease, multimorbidities, common behavioral comorbid conditions, and the need for behavioral interventions for lifestyle habits and behavioral conditions. In addition, trends in the industry toward value-based payment and the importance of integrated behavioral health in achieving value-based payment incentives should be emphasized [e.g., Kathol]. Here are examples of current trends and accompanying analyses for integrated behavioral health:

Your specific business and industry is integrated behavioral health, and the strategic opportunities include an increase in demand combined with a shortage of leaders and clinicians. The trends include increased hiring and associated needs that include, training, supervision, and performance management, all human resources issues.

An important organizing principle is the role of integrated behavioral health in achieving the Triple Aim of achieving improved patient experience of care, improved population health, and decreased cost of care (Berwick, Nolan, & Whittington, 2008), as well as the recent fourth dimension of provider stress and burnout (Bodenheimer & Sinsky, 2014).

Integrated behavioral health is part of the broader healthcare industry. In this section you should describe national, regional, and local healthcare industries and trends, especially those relevant to your integrated behavioral health program. National trends include government policy changes and updates. Examples include change in reimbursement, such as new value-based payment programs by CMS (Miller, Ross, Melek, Davis, & Kathol, 2017), and changes in healthcare policy, such as government changes that impact healthcare structure, reimbursement, etc.

This section should focus on your local healthcare industry and trends. Describe local hospitals, primary care, and community health centers, especially those relevant to your plan. Focus on payers, such as health plans, and their role in driving integrated behavioral health. Define the patient population in order to demonstrate the need for integrated care (e.g., chronic noncommunicable disease, obesity).

Describe the staging of integrated care maturity as new, expanding, or stable. Are there economic cycles or seasonal factors that can impact your plan?

Address regulation, licensure, certification, and accreditation relevant to your plan. What are key performance measures required by government and accreditation agencies, both national and local? What are health information technology changes such as electronic health records, interoperability, and meaningful use relevant to integrated care? What are financial issues relevant to integrated care? Examples include which reimbursement codes for integrated behavioral health in primary care settings are available in your area and which provider types are eligible for fee-for-service reimbursement. Are there emerging new payment models such as Accountable Care Organizations and/or value-based payment contracts relevant to your plan? What is the supply of eligible integrated behavioral health clinicians in your area, including license type and salary and benefit information?

Target Markets A comprehensive description and concise explanation of your target market will provide focus for your plan. This is your opportunity to share opportunities for integrated behavioral health with local leaders, payers, or potential investors to demonstrate your market potential. The first step is to show that you know your customers, who they are and what they want. The integrated behavioral health "customer" is diverse – payer, primary care physicians, CEO and CFO, and, of course, patients. The key customer is the target for reading the business plan that you hope to influence. However, covering all key customers/stakeholders will be of benefit to promote your plan. Describe how integrated behavioral health can improve patient and provider satisfaction, improve processes and efficiencies, improve clinical outcomes, and reduce high utilization and associated costs of care. The target market must be well-defined, meaningful, sizable, and easily reached, so describing how integrated behavioral health can benefit multiple customers.

Describe how integrated behavioral health can meet the interests and concerns of your customers. Define the patient market in terms of epidemiologic data on chronic disease, cardiometabolic risk factors, such as obesity, access to behavioral health, and satisfaction with healthcare. Describe the provider market by types of medical and behavioral providers, their perceived needs for integrated care. Ideally, complete a survey of provider interest and/or readiness for integrated behavioral health using surveys such as those found on the SAMHSA website: (ref). The market size and trends are likely to present opportunities to promote integrated behavioral health.

The Competition You must demonstrate a clear understanding of your competition for your business plan. This includes a critical self-assessment of your plan's strengths and weaknesses relative to competing programs. A SWOT analysis can be a useful exercise. What are the internal business resources that you will need to compete successfully?

Identify competing programs and evaluate how they are addressing the target market compared to your plan. Evaluate exactly what aspects of the market they compete with you. How does your plan compare to their services? What are potential future competitors that may emerge? What are barriers to entry in the market for you and competitors?

Describe your competitive position based on multiple factors that impact your potential for a successful integrated behavioral health program. What are the internal (e.g., personnel, finances) and external (e.g., current contracts or partners, reputation) strengths and weaknesses of your competitors? How are competitor services perceived by the different customer segments – providers, patients, and payers?

Identify other factors that can impact your competitive position such as first-to-market advantage. If you are first, how long before other competitors emerge in the market. Do you already have a base of operations, existing contracts or programs, to grow upon? How can you utilize the Internet to reduce barriers to entering the market? Most importantly, how can you distinguish your plan from the competition and what must the customer believe that they need from you so that they want your product?

Define the size of the market and the distribution of customers (patients, providers, healthcare systems, health plans) and how you will address a sufficient size of the market to sustain your product. Describe the barriers to entering the market, such as start-up costs, expert consultation, licensing or reimbursement problems, and market saturation.

Strategic Position and Risk Assessment Your strategic position defines exactly what your product is. It should include your product strengths and weaknesses and the context of industry trends, market changes, and competitive opportunities. The strategic position answers the question of why should customers buy your product? What are advantages that you offer to the competition? Your strategic position also defines areas that are out of the scope for your plan, in effect defining what you are not going to do in order to allocate resources effectively. Examples of strategic positions include customer perception, market segment and share, operational/technical advantages, propriety aspects of your product, sales and marketing, and your business model branding.

Risk assessment is critical to identify and reduce potential threats to your plan. Examples of risk include competing programs, changes in market, technology, execution, and finances. A SWOT analysis is an effective method of balancing risks and opportunities. The SWOT is a grid that defines the strengths, weaknesses, opportunities, and threats for your product.

Marketing Plan and Sales Strategy Marketing and sales are the core of the business plan in attracting buy-in from your target customer. Executives and investors evaluate marketing plans based on the ability to attract customers and provide a financial return. The resources required for marketing and sales must be cost-effective and sustainable in the context of your business finances. The typical behavioral entrepreneur will not have a traditional sales force at hand but may tap into existing organization resources and utilize cost-effective social media approaches to marketing.

The marketing plan must describe how you will communicate with and motivate your customers (executives, physicians, patients) to buy and use your product. The marketing plan is vital to a company's success because it illuminates the best way to communicate with, motivate, and secure customers. How will you disseminate this information in a cost-effective manner? Social media marketing approaches are ideal, combined with traditional approaches such as brochures, print media, and networking. Social media marketing approaches include using social media sites, blogs, podcasts, Twitter, LinkedIn, YouTube, mobile marketing, and email newsletters.

Your sales strategy must describe how you will achieve customer sales, staff responsible for sales strategies, and your sales process. How will you identify, outreach, meet, and follow-up with sales leads? In summary, this section must persuade your target customer that your plan will successfully contact customers, convince them to purchase your product, and be cost-effective.

Operations Operations are a critical component of integrated behavioral health business planning. How will your program be integrated within existing business operations in the case of an integrated behavioral health program in a primary care clinic? Operations include scheduling, workflows, procedures for hallway hand-off between the physician and behavioral consultant, assessment and intervention by the behavioral consultant, and follow-up activities. Careful planning in this area can result in improved productivity and cost savings while improving the quality of your product/service and enhancing the work environment for your employees. Your business operations must be tailored to the needs of the organization, perceived as desirable by customers, and not conflict with current business processes. Describe how your operations offer a competitive alternative to existing practices and overcome common barriers such as physician resistance.

In this section production refers to the key factors required to produce your product or services and associated costs. Integrated behavioral health production factors include behavioral health clinicians and their productivity, costs associated with screening and assessment, and implementing evidence-based practices (e.g., training, supervision). Record keeping, communications, and confidentiality procedures are important. Operations must also include the equivalent of inventory control, how you project the delivery of your services, in this case behavioral interventions for patients. In this context, your inventory is the patient population, and control is your description of how you will identify patient. Will this be by referral from PCP, by medical record diagnoses, or by high utilization and cost of care? What is the projected volume of patients, and how will you staff to meet the anticipated demand? How will your workflows incorporate the process improvement to maintain standard procedures?

Another component of operations is customer evaluation of the delivery and satisfaction with your product, including physicians and patients as stakeholders. A research component is also necessary to demonstrate clinical, quality, and ideally financial outcomes. Financial controls are necessary to insure you monitor costs and revenue to ensure profitability and sustainability.

Technology Plan In the technology section, you must describe how your integrated behavioral health program will integrated with the existing practice health information technology, as well as any new health technologies that are a component of your plan. Health information technology includes the electronic medical record (EMR), billing and claims, a patient registry, patient portal, remote telemedicine, online screening and assessment, and increasingly mHealth apps and wearable sensors. You must demonstrate an understanding of how your plan will meet the organization technology needs. If you have new technologies, you must explain how they will be integrated.

This section is also an opportunity to highlight the benefits of your plan based on health technology. How will you utilize health technology to achieve the triple aim? Will you incorporate existing or add new online screening for behavioral health? Will you use a patient registry as a component of a population health management program for patients with comorbid type 2 diabetes and depression? Will you incorporate mHealth apps and wearable sensors in for nutrition, physical activity, etc., in your behavioral interventions? You must demonstrate adequate planning of both technology and cost issues associated with your plan.

Management and Organization In this section describe your management team and your management style. Your reader will carefully evaluate the background of key employees. If you have your own company describe the board of directors, advisory committee, consultants or contractors. Describe the credentials and responsibilities for key team members and the compensation and benefits package. Your management structure includes the organization structure, the lines of reporting, supervision, and training. Your management style includes both formal and informal approaches to managing employee performance.

Social Responsibility and Sustainability In this section demonstrate integrity and corporate citizenship. Social responsibility demonstrates your commitment to the organization, the community, and the economy. For integrated behavioral health programs, ethics, privacy, and confidentiality are important. Interprofessional team building and teamwork are also highly relevant. Concern for the environment is also beneficial. Demonstrating strong social responsibility will be attractive both to your target customer but also contribute to recruiting new employees. Social ventures invent something, bring something to market, create new services, provide services, and adapt an existing product.

Development, Milestones, and Exit Plan In this describe the anticipated growth of your company over time, milestones you will achieve, and if appropriate an exit strategy. Describe your vision of where your company will be in terms of milestones at the end of year 1, 3, and 5. Define long-term goals in objective terms. What is your business strategy and what are your priorities? What are recent milestones and what are current activities designed to achieve strategic initiatives?

What are potential risks to your business model and how can you evaluate them and use scenario testing to demonstrate your ability to respond to adverse business situations? An exit plan is appropriate for a business or product that is designed with the intention of a buyout, acquisition, sale, merger, etc.

The Financials This section will consist of your financial projections for the business case using a pro forma to document program costs and revenue. The pro forma includes your income, cash flow, and balance sheet on an annual basis. Include financial data for recent years in an existing program and for 3 to 5 years into the future. Define your financial assumptions, such as costs for salary and benefit package for behavioral health consultants, projected revenue based on billing, claims, and reimbursement. Your financials should be conservative, honest, and consistent with industry practice. Key sections of the financials include: staffing, cash flow projections, income statements, a balance sheet, how funds are used, a break-even analysis, and a financial assumptions section.

The Appendix The appendix is used for documents that are too detailed or lengthy to be included in the sections of your business plan. Use the appendix to demonstrate attention to detail that is relevant to your target audience for the plan. Examples of information appropriate for an integrated behavioral health appendix include market research, resumes for key personnel, screening and assessment measures, behavioral intervention protocols, and technology information.

Case Example: Behavioral Health Entrepreneurship Course

An exemplar course for integrated behavioral health is the Behavioral Health Entrepreneurship course offered in the Arizona State University, Doctor of Behavioral Health degree program. This is an online course delivered in 8 weeks, a one-half semester course that contains the equivalent content of a full 15-week semester course (see Appendix). The course includes asynchronous content such as discussion board questions and replies, reading assignments, links to relevant web sites or YouTube digital media, and written assignments. In addition, the course includes synchronous content in the form of a weekly live class Webinar for discussion and two group activities that are conducted by groups of four to six students using an online videoconference platform. Students are expected to spend 15–18 hours per week in readings, assignments, and related activities. The course learning objectives are:

1. Evaluate and explain the range of entrepreneurial opportunities open to behavioral health clinicians.
2. Develop a specific entrepreneurial concept based on this evaluation of entrepreneurial opportunities.
3. Develop steps and identify resources needed for a start-up business.

4. Create a formal business plan for an integrated medical and behavioral healthcare program.
5. Create strategies to demonstrate the value of a behavioral health clinician in a medical setting with strategies to promote clinical identity in the medical setting.
6. Compose a plan to speak with upper management in healthcare regarding the behavioral care provider's skillset and ability to provide process improvements to their business.

The key assignment in the class is to write an integrated behavioral health business plan. The written business plan assignment is divided into two sections. In addition, the students develop a PowerPoint slide presentation designed for a business pitch. Students use one group activity to meet and present a draft of their business plan pitch using the PowerPoint slides. The group activity is structured as a role-play with the student presenting to student peers who play the role of stakeholders for the proposal. The actual PowerPoint pitch is recorded online and viewed and graded by the instructor. The group activity is structured as a role-play with the student presenting to student peers who play the role of stakeholders for the proposal. The grading rubrics will be covered in the next section as examples of measuring core competencies for the integrated behavioral health entrepreneur.

Measurement of Effective Behavioral Entrepreneurship Training

This section contains descriptions of assignments from the Behavioral Health Entrepreneurship course described above, including grading rubric sections to demonstrate approaches to measurement of competencies for writing and presenting an integrated behavioral health business plan. While these examples are from an online course, that same content may be delivered in an in-person course or seminar. The first key competency is writing a business plan, a complex task that will be novel to most physicians and behavioral consultants. Sufficient time must be provided for the student to write the plan with feedback. A second key competency is to create a PowerPoint presentation based on the plan and make a verbal pitch for the proposal. It is highly recommended that both the written and verbal presentation are included in any course for behavioral entrepreneurship.

Discussion of key topics is helpful for students to demonstrate competencies in achieving learning objectives and as a means of inquiry and feedback to peer students and the instructor. Each student writes a reply to the question posted by the instructor and then writes a reply to the post of at least one other student post. Here is a sample discussion question from the course:

Discussion Board Assignment

The focus of the assigned readings this week is strategic planning and management. For this discussion board, you are to complete a SWOT analysis based on a current situation in your place of employment or if you are not currently employed based on a case scenario of launching and integrated behavioral health program in a primary care clinic. Consider the clinical, operational, and financial strategies for the design of your integrated behavioral health program. List a minimum of two to three strengths, weaknesses, opportunities, and threats for the topic that you pick. Use the SWOT analysis to help guide your strategic planning for the written business plan assignment. In addition to these instructions, the course includes links to guidelines for writing a SWOT analysis, as well as YouTube video tutorials, and written examples.

The written business plan and PowerPoint presentation assignments are based on the 13 components of a business plan in the course textbook by Abrams (2014). The instructor provides detailed feedback on each paper, with suggestions for improvement and questions if necessary. The instructor applies a grading rubric for each component of the assignment. The grading rubric for these assignments is too long to be shown here in their entirety; however, sample competencies from assignment 1 are listed in the table below, along with how each is measured.

The PowerPoint business plan pitch is recorded using the VoiceThread online resource, reviewed and graded by the instructor. The grading rubric sections include content design of the slides, the content of the business plan, the verbal delivery and presentation, and the delivery organization. The instructor provides written feedback to the student and applies the grading rubric for each component of the assignment.

Summary The current state of healthcare transformation demands that the integrated behavioral health leader develops competencies as a business entrepreneur. The Triple Aim focuses on improved patient experience of care, population health, and cost savings which require business acumen to balance clinical and cost outcomes. The transition from fee-for-service to value-based healthcare will demand leaders who can effectively promote and negotiate innovative approaches to reimbursement for integrated behavioral health services. Most leaders in integrated behavioral health do not have formal education and training on business entrepreneurship, leaving them ill-prepared to address these new challenges. Developing an effective business plan is a key component of successful entrepreneurship. Specific training strategies and techniques are needed to help the learner acquire core skills and competencies necessary for developing an integrated behavioral health business plan. Developing these competencies will contribute to raising awareness of healthcare executives to the importance of integrated behavioral health in the emerging world of value-based primary healthcare delivery.

Appendix: Behavioral Health Entrepreneurship Course Calendar

Arizona State University Doctor of Behavioral Health Program

Week	Topics/lessons	Activities	Assignments
1	Introduction to course and assignments Introduction to successful business plan: starting the process and components	Read: Syllabus Read: Abrams Ch. 1–5 Read: Christensen Ch. 1	Classmate introduction post (no points) Introduction post due Sunday by 11:59pm (AZ time) Discussion board #1Initial post due Friday by 11:59pm AZ time Reply post due Sunday by 11:59pm (AZ time)
2	Successful business plan components Disruption in business Introduction to getting entrepreneurial: mission: customer/ product, innovationBCP opportunities in integrated care *Weekly Webinar*: Tuesday at 4:00 pm AZ time	Read: Abrams 6–10 Read: Christensen, Ch. 2 Read Farrell Ch. 1–3 Watch videos embedded in week 1 course content Attend Webinar or watch Webinar recording	Discussion board #2 Initial post due Friday by 11:59pm AZ time Reply post due Sunday by 11:59pm (AZ time)
3	Successful business plan components Disruptive innovation Getting entrepreneurial: self-inspired Behavior: What's really required? Assignment #1 business plan outline *Weekly Webinar*: Tuesday at 4:00 pm AZ time	Read: Abrams 11–17 Read: Christensen, Ch. 3 Read: Farrell, Ch. 4, Conclusion Watch videos embedded in week 2 course content Attend Webinar or watch Webinar recording	Discussion board #3 Initial post due Friday by 11:59pm AZ time Reply post due Sunday by 11:59pm (AZ time) Assignment #1: *Business plan part 1* Due: Sunday by 11:59pm (AZ time)
4	Successful business plan: putting the plan to work Clinical financial analysis *Weekly Webinar:* Tuesday at 4:00 pm AZ time	Read: Abrams Ch. 18–22 Read: Christensen, Ch.4 Watch videos embedded in week 3 course content Attend Webinar or watch Webinar recording	Learning Assessment #1: Due: Sunday by 11:59pm (AZ time)

Week	Topics/lessons	Activities	Assignments
5	Business plan development (continued) Billing systems and projections *Weekly Webinar:* Tuesday at 4:00 pm AZ time	Read: Ries, Ch.1–4 Read: Christensen, Ch.7 Watch videos embedded in week 4 course content Attend Webinar or watch Webinar recording	Assignment #2: *Business plan part 2* Due: Sunday by 11:59pm (AZ time)
6	Formatting of business plan, review of any questions and answers Sample business plans Issues facing integrated care ventures *Weekly Webinar:* Tuesday at 4:00 pm AZ time	Read: Ries, Ch., 5–8 Read: Christensen, Ch. 11 Watch videos embedded in week 5 course content Attend Webinar or watch Webinar recording	Team activity (Due Sunday 11:59 PM AZ time) Learning assessment #2: Due: Sunday by 11:59pm (AZ time)
7	PowerPoint pitch overviewReading/ videos discussion Preparing for the workforce *Weekly Webinar:* Thursday at 4:00 pm AZ time	Read: Ries, Ch. 13–14 Watch videos embedded in week 5 course content Attend Webinar or watch Webinar recording	Assignment #3 - *PPT pitch* Due Sunday 11:59 PM (AZ time) Discussion board #4Initial post due Friday by 11:59pm AZ time Reply post due Sunday by 11:59pm (AZ time)
Wrap-Up	Case study in integrated care entrepreneurship *Final Weekly Webinar:* Tuesday at 4:00 pm AZ time	No Readings Watch videos embedded in week 7 course content Attend Final Webinar or watch Webinar recording Develop PPT and post DB #5	No assignments due

References

Abrams, R. (2014). *Successful business plan: Secrets, & strategies*. Palo Alto, CA: Planning Shop.

Berwick, D., Nolan, T., & Whittington, J. (2008). The triple aim: Care, health, and cost. *Health Affairs, 27*(3), 759–769. https://doi.org/10.1377/hlthaff.27.3.759.

Bodenheimer, T., & Sinsky, C. (2014). From triple to quadruple aim: Care of the patient requires care of the provider. *Annals of Family Medicine, 12*(6), 573–576. https://doi.org/10.1370/afm.1713.

Boore, J., and Porter, S. (2011) Education for entrepreneurship in nursing. *Nurse Education Today, 31*(2):18–191.

CCSE, Social entrepreneurship discussion paper no. 1. Alberta, Canada: Canadian Centre for Social Entrepreneurship, Duke University: The Fuqua School of Business. (2001).

Cohn, K., and Schwartz, R. (2002). Business plan writing for physicians. *Am J Surg, 182*(4):11–120.

Miller, B., Ross, K., Melek, S., Davis, M., & Kathol, R. (2017). Payment reform in the patient-centered medical home: Enabling and sustaining integrated behavioral health care. *American Psychologist, 72*(1), 55–68.

NICENT Entrepreneurship awareness — an elearning moduleUniversity of Ulster, NICENT (2004).

Shatz, T., Shatz, I., Becker, S., Patel, J., and Eysenbach. (2014) Promoting business and entrepreneurial awareness in health care professionals: lessons from venture capital panels at Medicine 2.0 conferences. *J Med Internet Res, 16*(8):e184 https://doi.org/10.2196/jmir.3390.

Chapter 9
Graduate Internship Training of Integrated Behavioral Health in Primary Care (IBHPC)

C. R. Macchi and Colleen Clemency Cordes

Chapter overview	
Domains	*Training programs* *Workforce development* *BHP skill development* *Evidence-based practice* *Three worlds of healthcare service delivery* *Interprofessional education*
Key points	*Focused training programs* *Prevention, treatment, and support of healthy patient behaviors* *Continuous monitoring and evaluating of provider skills refinement* *Address clinical, operational, and financial activities of team-based care delivery* *Incorporate multi-observer, multi-rater evaluation processes*
Foundational knowledge and skills	*Targeted training and refinement of specific BHP skills* *Communication* *Problem-solving* *Team collaboration* *Patient engagement*
Student learning objectives (SLOs)	*Learners will:* *Identify targeted performance indicators and related behavioral anchors* *Focus skill refinement practice management, patient engagement, and team-based activities*
Instructional strategies	*Training and assessment planning template* *Asynchronous online learning modules* *In-person, flipped classroom*

C. R. Macchi (✉) · C. C. Cordes
Integrated Behavioral Health Programs, College of Health Solutions, Arizona State University, Phoenix, AZ, USA
e-mail: crmacchi@asu.edu; Colleen.Clemency@asu.edu

C. R. Macchi, R. Kessler (eds.), *Training to Deliver Integrated Care*,
https://doi.org/10.1007/978-3-319-78850-0_9

Chapter overview	
Evaluating learning	*BHP Performance Evaluation Tool* *Multilevel monitoring and measuring of metrics and/or outcomes* *Practitioner* *Integrate care team* *Patient* *Healthcare delivery system* *Multi-observer, multi-rater evaluation processes*

Historical/Traditional Approaches to Internship Training

Given the differentiation of skills necessary for the behavioral health provider (BHP) working in integrated primary care versus specialty mental health, the need to train and/or retrain behavioral health providers to work in primary care has been evident for some time. Initial efforts at training, such providers began almost 25 years ago, with the establishment of a postdoctoral fellowship for psychologists at the University of Rochester Medical Center Family Medicine Residency Program (S. McDaniel, personal communication). Designed to provide psychologists with the requisite training to fill both clinical and academic roles as behavioral scientists in family medicine, the program focused (and continues to focus) on the role of psychologists as members of the primary care team using family psychology and systems theory training approaches (https://www.urmc.rochester.edu/psychiatry/education/training/post-doctoral/primary-care.aspx). This program, and clinical health psychology postdoctoral fellowships that subsequently emerged, offered psychologists the opportunity to gain hands-on training in primary care psychology under the direct supervision of licensed psychologists. The in-person training paradigm, which subsequently expanded to predoctoral internship rotations and experiences in primary care, remained the predominant approach for exposure to and training in team-based primary care for almost 20 years, with the American Psychological Association (APA) accrediting its first clinical health psychology fellowship at Michigan State/Flint Area Medical Education in 1999. Despite the growth and expansion of such hands-on training experiences, only 11% of APA-accredited psychology programs offer some sort of training in primary care psychology (American Psychological Association Education Directorate, n.d.), and only 33% of predoctoral internships offer a similar experience (appic.org).

Beginning in the mid-2000s, the need for additional post-professional retraining experiences became evident, as the demand for integrated behavioral providers exceeded the availability of trained providers (Blount & Miller, 2009; Hall et al., 2015). The need for additional on-the-job training, coupled with research suggesting that online training modalities can produce as positive learning outcomes as in-person training (Means, Toyama, Murphy, Bakia, & Jones, 2009), resulted in the emergence of a number of Internet-based training options. In 2007, the University of Massachusetts Medical School launched the first CE-based certificate program in integrated primary care; the following decade saw expansion of programming in similar continuing education, the expansion of professional organizations (e.g., the Collaborative Family Healthcare Association; cfha.net) and related programming and interprofessional training initiatives (American Psychological Association, Interprofessional Seminar on Integrated Primary Care Work Group, 2016). More about training and workforce development training initiatives will be discussed in Chap. 11. By 2009, Arizona State University's Doctor of Behavioral Health Program (chs.asu.edu/dbh) emerged to exclusively focus on graduate-level training of integrated behavioral health clinicians and managers on the clinical, financial, and operational domains of integrated primary care.

Despite the increase in training opportunities, there remain significant shortages in the IBH workforce. Organizations frequently struggle to hire, train, and retain qualified professionals (Hall et al., 2015). It is clear that training capacity does not currently meet the workforce demands (Hall et al., 2015; Serrano, Cordes, Cubic, & Daub, 2017) and that there remains a need for the field to coalesce around a single, unifying set of competencies. From 2014 to 2016, competencies for practice in integrated primary care were put forth both by guild-specific organizations (e.g., American Psychological Association, 2015), government-sponsored organizations (Hoge, Morris, Laraia, Pomerantz, & Farley, 2014), policy centers (Miller et al., 2016), and others. While significant similarities exist across these competencies, such as interprofessional collaboration and a focus on systems-oriented, evidence-based practice, these competencies are more limited in their attention to the operational and financial knowledge, skills, and abilities that are essential to the sustainability of an integrated primary care program (see Chap. 3).

Key Conceptual and Operational Shifts

Training programs and initiatives began with the intent of preparing behavioral practitioners to work in primary care settings (Blount & Miller, 2009). While innovative, the efforts to integrate BH in primary care have often been guided by the assumption that everything else within the practice may remain the same. Increasingly, the insertion of a BHP into primary care had been met with medical team concern about the potential disruptions of existing workflows or team preference to simply refer patients with mental health issues to a BHP who operated in a separate physical space within or outside of the clinic that offered traditional psychotherapy and had separate clinical records separate from the medical records. As a result, early training was focused primarily on preparing BHPs to enter an unfamiliar medical environment with limited integrated operations.

Medical and mental/behavioral health focuses training that targets prevention, treatment, and support of healthy patient behaviors. Behavior is a common factor that is related to each dimension of patients' biopsychosocial health (i.e., medical, mental health, and relational issues), general functioning, and overall well-being. Cognitions and emotions play a vital role in patients' perceptions and decision-making abilities. Focusing primarily on health behaviors provides an observable and measureable way to target patients' health behavior change efforts. Training in integrated behavioral health practice highlights patient health behaviors as a common factor that coalesces when medical and behavioral health providers work together to provide comprehensive, collaborative health care services.

As integrated behavioral healthcare has developed, training objectives and strategies have progressively shifted to focus healthcare delivery to operationalize a biopsychosocial approach to care (Baird, Hepworth, Myerholtz, & Reitz, 2017). An integrated, patient-centered approach requires retraining for each member of the integrated care team that facilitates operational adjustments. Increasingly, each team member is trained to address varying levels of patients' BH issues within the exam room with varied results (Hall et al., 2015; Martin, 2017). This team-based approach requires each member to be aware of and address each of the three worlds of healthcare delivery (i.e., clinical, operational, financial) and to consider the interdependence of practices within each world with the other two (Peek, 2008).

The clinical world of practice requires training programs that are focused on improving each team member's medical and/or behavioral literacy and the use of brief, evidence-based, behavioral assessments and interventions. Behavioral practitioners learn about patients' common medical conditions, processes, and treatments, while medical practitioners learn about patients' common behavioral issues related to specific medical conditions. Each team member is trained to develop the skills needed to use broad-based assessments that are sensitive enough to detect med/BH comorbidities. Training presents the complementarity of medical and behavioral interventions and treatments that effectively address patients' use of self-management activities and reduce suffering (Egnew, 2017). Training programs address the operational world by presenting the implications of care planning, delivery, and evaluation on workflows and team-based integrated, coordinated, and collaborative care. All team members are trained to understand and employ quality improvement practices that guide continuous practice innovations, assessments, and refinements and facilitate iterative, care delivery improvement processes. Training components that focus on the financial world examine ways to reduce costs and improve efficiencies of clinical and operational practices. Training that targets the financial world improves team members' awareness and consideration of treatment costs and available payment options.

Consider a few examples that illustrate the implications of relationships of each world on the "other two worlds" with a range of training objectives (Peek, 2008):

- Teams striving to accomplish the Triple Aim (IHI, 2015) work to expand preventative programs and services that address patients' conditions earlier in the disease process.

  - Clinical – improve patient health outcomes
  - Operational – provide alternative services
  - Financial – fewer chronic patients lead to less cost

- Training that improves monitoring of the returns on investment (ROI) associated with service and program changes enables those teams to simultaneously strive toward improving health outcomes while searching for increasingly efficient practices.
  - Clinical – improve patient health outcomes
  - Operational – improve service and/or program delivery
  - Financial – increase return on investment (ROI)

- Team members are trained to be more aware of and responsive to evolving policies and practices and to use team-based productivity metrics as a basis for identifying and targeting opportunities to change care coordination and collaborations.
  - Clinical – improve patient satisfaction with health care services
  - Operational – develop care coordination and collaboration processes; increase team productivity
  - Financial – decrease cost of labor for the existing services provided

Training Barriers

There is an adage that "you can't teach an old dog new tricks," and leaders in the world of integrated care have certainly argued that this holds true with regard to the professional development of integrated behavioral health providers (Serrano, 2015). Given this and that there exists a significant workforce shortage for the provision of integrated primary care behavioral health, leaders in the field have increasingly called upon graduate training programs to enhance their preprofessional training opportunities in integrated primary care behavioral health (Blount & Miller, 2009). Despite the diversity of training backgrounds among integrated behavioral health providers (e.g., psychologists, social workers, counselors, marriage, and family therapists), most efforts to date to infuse graduate programs with IBH curricula have been guild-specific (Serrano et al., 2017). Such siloed approaches to training are often a function of the need to adhere to secondary accreditation standards; however, these restrictions often inadvertently result in a student's view of patient concerns from a single perspective: that of a mental health provider. When learners are unwilling or unable to transition their schema of patient care to team-based, holistic care, challenges in professional role delineation and scope of practice emerge. Given the nature of primary care and the ramifications of a siloed worldview on primary care integration (e.g., provision of colocated specialty mental health services rather than integrated care), there is a need to train to the realities of such team-based collaborative approaches.

Interprofessional education (IPE) has emerged as a promising educational approach that allows for concurrent and collaborative training across professional disciplines (Reeves, Palaganas, & Zierler, 2017); however, many of these training opportunities occur either at the undergraduate or post-professional stage or are limited to academic medical settings (Curran et al., 2012; Cubic, Mance, Turgesen, & Lamanna, 2012). Interprofessional education actively engages trainees from diverse disciplines (e.g., mental health, nursing, pharmacy, medicine) to work together to solve complex cases; such training gives students an opportunity to understand the perspectives of different disciplines and promote team-based collaboration. While promising, a recent review of the literature reviewed that positive outcomes from IPE have focused primarily on learner's knowledge acquisition and attitudes toward collaboration; little attention has been paid to individual behavior change or organizational change to promote collaboration (Reeves et al., 2017; Cubic et al., 2012).

As noted above, historical siloed training approaches may, in part, be a function of secondary accreditation standards that promote generalist training and may be rigid in their instructional delivery (Serrano et al., 2017). There have been notable efforts to infuse integrated care curricula into traditional mental health programming, such as the American Psychological Association's (APA) development of "plug-and-play" curriculum on integrated primary care, which is a freely available resource consisting of four 120-min modules and can be readily infused into existing coursework by graduate programs (Society for Health Psychology, 2018).

Acknowledging that the provision of integrated primary care behavioral health training may be difficult for the faculty who lack practical experience in that environment and may come from a traditional mental health background and mindset, the committee on integrated primary care within the APA are providing consultation and mentoring to graduate faculty who chose to adopt the curricula (Society for Health Psychology, 2018). Similarly, the Social Work and Integrated Behavioral Healthcare Project began in 2012, with the focus on developing curricula revolving around clinical practice and policy and services (www.csew.org) for use in social work graduate programs. These predeveloped training modules, along with other widely available asynchronous training modules, may be one approach to infusing curricula into programs with limited time for additional coursework. Flipped classroom approaches and/or asynchronous learning opportunities within the graduate training experience may assist in enhancing preprofessional knowledge and skill development.

Training or Skill Acquisition

Previous chapters addressed skills unique to each content area such as team-based strategies (Chap. 3), population-based approaches to patient health management (Chap. 4), and healthcare management practices (Chap. 7). Each of these key areas supports an integrated approach to providing effective patient-centered care. Effective training programs must incorporate activities to support and performance metrics to monitor learner skill development. Training activities should focus on crosscutting skills coupled with opportunities to perform specific team-based activities, as pedagogical approaches are increasingly moving away from didactic, knowledge-based learning instructor-led lectures and information transmission (Malott, Hall, Sheely-Moore, Krell, & Cardaciotto, 2014). Instead, new approaches are offering learners with varied opportunities to engage in active learning experiences that actively process and apply information while developing communication and problem-solving and adjust to timely feedback from their peers and instructors (Wieman, 2014).

Measurement

Training approaches should be designed to monitor and respond to changes in performance metrics that address each of the following four levels:

1. Practitioner performance – a practitioner's performance in team-based care with a range of patients
2. Integrated care team performance – a team of practitioners' engagement in clinical workflows and coordination of patient care
3. Patient outcomes – the impact of team-based care on improving patient health outcomes
4. Healthcare delivery system performance – the medical team and healthcare managers demonstration of improving patient satisfaction and health outcomes while improving efficiency of healthcare delivery and reducing costs

Establishing a valid, reliable performance measurement begins with identifying what to measure followed by anticipating and interpreting the potential results of the data (Macchi et al., 2016). This training manual places an emphasis on the first level of practitioner competency-based training approaches that explicitly target expected outcomes or competencies. Reliable metrics require establishing observable, behavioral evidences for each competency, often referred to as behavioral anchors. Varied raters should be able to use the anchors as a lens to observe the learner's performance and apply consistent ratings of each competency. One more useful guide is to provide additional contextual information about where to look for specific behaviors reflecting each competency.

Performance Evaluation The *BHP performance evaluation tool* was developed to assess BHP knowledge and application related to four domains of skills (Macchi, 2016): (1) conceptual and professional development, (2) clinical skills and practice, (3) practice management, and (4) demonstrated awareness of financial management. An analysis of existing lists of core competencies from the APA

Interorganizational Workgroup (APA, 2015), SAMHSA-HRSA Center for Integrated Health Solutions (Hoge et al., 2014), AHRQ Academy (Kinman, Gilchrist, Payne-Murphy, & Miller, 2015), Colorado Consensus Conference Report (Miller et al., 2016), and Robinson and Reiter (2015) revealed clusters of common skills reflected in each of the first three domains. The fourth domain emerged from key themes reflected in the three worlds model of healthcare (Peek, 2008). Several key integrated healthcare leaders reviewed and provided feedback throughout the development and refinement of the evaluation tool.

Table 9.1 provides a snapshot of several items that measure the conceptual and professional development domain. The first 20 knowledge or skill items on the performance evaluation tool are evaluated on two practice delivery dimensions: clinical and operational (i.e., marked with C or O, respectively) applications. These two dimensions are intended to determine the levels at which a BHP performs clinical and related operational activities that are intended to support the item. An observer, usually a preceptor or other medical team member, scores each dimension using the following criteria: proficient, progressing, missing, and not observed. The proficient response suggests that the learner has reached a level of consistent mastery. The progressing option suggests that the learner still has room for growth and development and often reflects inconsistent performance in the identified area. The missing response suggests that there has been no observable evidence of performance during occasions when the observer would expect to have seen the related behaviors. The not observed response suggests that the observer was not present to observe the learner's behavior.

The items that address the BHP's conceptual and professional development are listed in the first column (i.e., systems orientation, primary care culture, cultural adaptation, professionalism, practice-based learning). Each item is further divided into related clinical and operational dimensions (see cultural adaptation, items 5 and 6). Measurement targets the degree to which the BHP demonstrates performing the behavioral anchors (third column) related to the BHP's clinical approach to perform warm handoffs and the extent to which the BHP addresses the operational process of collaborating with the other medical team members. For each item, the tool provides the rater with the focus of evaluation, or context, where the behavior may be observed in practice (fourth column). In this case, the BHP would be observed to be available to provide patients with immediate BH assistance during an office visit with another provider, and other team members would report on their collaborations with the BHP and the BHP's demonstrated support of shared team goals. Using a detailed evaluation tool enables the trainer to develop programs that target specific competencies. Subsequent to providing the BHP training, the trainer could use the tool to measure the BHP's demonstrated evidence of those competencies in practice over time. While the tool provides global measurements of observed behaviors, an additional set of performance metrics is needed to monitor incremental, daily activities.

Table 9.1 Sample of BHP performance evaluation tool – conceptual and professional development domain

	Knowledge or skill	Dimensions	Care behavioral anchors	Focus of evaluation	Proficient	Progressing	Missing	Not observed
Conceptual & Professional Development								
1	Systems orientation	C	Identifies clinical models that are appropriate for the primary care setting	Verbal report to mentor includes description of approach among range of models				
2		O	Identifies policies and procedures related to sustaining integrated practices	Refers to related on-site policies in descriptions of clinical practices				
3	Primary care culture	C	Communicates unique features of primary care setting	Suggests clinical approaches that work well within primary care setting				
4		O	Practices brief hallway consultations with other clinic providers	Review of occurrences of hallway handoffs				
5	Cultural adaptation	C	Readily available for warm handoffs during patient exam visits	Available to provide patients with immediate BH assistance				
6		O	Collaboration with medical team performance	Feedback from medical team reports about intern support of medical team goals				
7	Professionalism	C	Clearly describes the unique, complimentary roles of each member of the interprofessional medical team	Performs a unique clinical role on interprofessional medical team				
8		O	Collaborates well with other providers in the clinic	Medical team feedback about student intern collaborative interactions				

(continued)

Table 9.1 (continued)

	Knowledge or skill	Dimensions	Care behavioral anchors	Focus of evaluation	Proficient	Progressing	Missing	Not observed
9	Practice-based Learning	C	Generates educational opportunities for practice members to examine behavioral factors related to patient medical conditions, (e.g., lunch and learns)	Review list of presentations student intern shared with medical team				

Item evaluation scale (Select ☒ the column that applies to each item)
Proficient – The student intern ***consistently demonstrates*** behaviors that are appropriate and applicable to the current work
Progressing – The student intern ***occasionally demonstrates*** behaviors that are appropriate and applicable to the current work
Missing – The student intern ***does not demonstrate*** behaviors when it would be appropriate and applicable to the current work
Not observed – The student ***has not had the opportunity*** for the evaluator to observe the student's behavior

Table 9.2 BHP performance metrics and targets

Categories	Metric	Description of assessment	Example target
Time with patients	% of clinic time in direct-patient contact	Assesses BHP's availability to see patients within the clinic	Minimum of 80% of total time in clinic
	Average time with patients	Assesses the degree to which the BHP's patient care fits with the clinic workflow	Maximum average of 30 min per patient visit
Outcome monitoring	% of patients administered validated outcome measures – initial and follow-up visits	Assesses the BHP's monitoring of patient outcomes over time	Minimum of 65% of all patient visits
	Average number of measures administered per patient	Assesses the BHP's refinement of clinical judgment skills needed to choose the right measure for the patient within a specific visit	Average of one validated measure for each patient
Patient engagement	% of patients referred to self-management resources	Assesses the BHP's attention to patients' use of self-management resources between office visits	Minimum of 25% of all patient visits
Team collaboration	Average number of warm handoffs	Assesses inclusion of BHP's services as part of integrated team	Minimum of 50% of all patient visits
	% of initial visits discussed with the PCP face-to-face	Assesses BHP's communication with PCP to coordinate care	Minimum of 75% of all patient visits
	% of scheduled patient visits separate from PCP visit	Assesses clinic's inclusion of BHP's services as part of integrated team	Maximum of 25% of all patient visits
	% of scheduled appointments	Assesses BHP's availability for warm handoffs and team consultations	Maximum of 50% of all patient visits

Performance Metrics An additional set of performance metrics provides a way to quantitatively measure activities specific to the role of the BHP on the medical team. The data associated with BHP-related activities within team-based integrated care environments are then compared with performance targets (see Table 9.2). Currently, there is a paucity of data to suggest standard BHP performance targets. Depending upon the type of clinical setting, initial targets may be set and then revised as the level of practice integration changes, and the BHP becomes more integrated into the clinic workflows. Within specific clinical settings, trainers and healthcare managers are likely to combine these metrics with the data from other measurements to assess the potential effects varied BHP activities on team collaboration efforts, patient access and outcomes, quality of care, finances, and healthcare system processes.

The metrics assess four broad categories of BHP activities: time with patients, monitoring outcomes, patient engagement in care, and collaborating with the integrated care team. Since there is little evidence to support targets (except as cited), those listed are currently inferred from available sources addressing key components of integrated related care or process outcome measures (SAMHSA-HRSA, 2014). Monitoring the BHP's time in direct-patient contacts reveals the BHP's availability to see patients within the clinic. This availability is dependent upon providing targeted, effective care with those patients. Monitoring the length of patient visits assesses the BHP's efficient use of time while gauging the degree to which the BHP's patient care fits within the clinic workflow. Data associated with the BHP's use of validated outcome measures addresses important issues related to the BHP's ability to use data to target interventions and expected patient outcomes. Those who effectively target patient interventions must develop the clinical judgment to determine the most appropriate validated measure for that patient in that visit then to use that data to monitor a patient's health status over time. Monitoring the number of patient referrals to self-management resources assesses the BHP's efforts to increase patient awareness and encouraging the use of self-management resources between office visits. Additional metrics have been suggested to further assess the BHP's availability to and work with the medical team, including number of handoffs, scheduled visits with PCP, and scheduled visits separate from PCP.

Example Template for Developing a Training Program

Most multifaceted evaluation tools can be used to establish a per item and overall assessment baseline. Data that reveal deficits on specific items could provide the focus for developing and offering learners with training programs that target areas of need. As a follow-up assessment, the tool could be readministered to assess changes in provider performance on the same targeted areas. Another section of the *BHP performance evaluation tool* (see Table 9.3) provides areas of focused assessment, training development, and reassessment of practice management skills.

The following training and assessment planning template addresses three targeted practice management skills (see Table 9.4). Working from left to right, the trainer gathers data using the performance evaluation tool that reflects progressing or missing ratings for the targeted items and identifies specific behavioral anchors associated with the rating for each item. The trainer would determine the appropriate performance metrics that would best reflect and quantify the BHP's skills and use the metric to establish a baseline rating for each (see italicized items as examples). Data gathered for each metric may occur through direct observation of the BHP's activities and/or interviewing team members working most closely with the learners. Next, the trainer would identify specific training strategies that would be

Table 9.3 Sample of BHP performance evaluation tool – practice management domain

Practice management				
23	Documentation	C	Develops clinical notes that provide a clear and succinct summary of patient BH issues directly related to medical condition(s)	Review clarity and form of student intern's clinical notes
24		O	Develops clear, accurate EHR notes that are understandable and useful to other medical team members	Review applicability of student intern's clinical notes to other team members' roles
25	Time management	C	Performs brief, targeted patient assessments and interventions	Student intern's visits with patients average less than 30 min
26		O	Work with patients supports the established clinic workflow	Feedback from medical director and other medical team members of student intern's participation in workflows
27	Resource management	C	Appropriately refers patients to self-management and/or community resources with clear rationale for referral	Review the relevance of the list of resources referred to patient conditions and needs
28		O	Appropriately refers patients to other medical learn members with clear rationale for referral	Feedback from medical team that intern provides appropriate referrals
29	Compliance with clinic policies and protocols	C	Uses approaches to patient care that are consistent with clinic policies	Feedback from team lead that intern supports clinic policies and procedures
30		O	Demonstrates support of existing clinic workflows and practices	Feedback from medical team that intern supports practices

used to develop and implement a targeted training program. Upon completion of the program, the trainer would administer the performance evaluation tool and rate the BHP's demonstrated skills using each metric. An analysis comparing baseline and follow-up data would assist with determining the need for additional training on the same skills or other skills.

The training template can be used to focus and plan training programs and evaluate learner performance on a range of clinical activities. The use of the template can also assist the trainer with the incremental process of refining behavioral anchors, performance metric targets, and team-feedback mechanisms. As the trainer refines these evaluation tools, additional analyses of the associations between learner performance adjustments and other clinic metrics (e.g., patient satisfaction, patient health outcomes) could further inform the development of training programs.

Table 9.4 Sample training and assessment planning template

Planning and baseline measurements				Training design and implementation	Follow-up measurements	
Baseline assessment	Targeted skills	Performance goals (Behavioral anchors)	Baseline metric	Training priorities	Assessment	Metric
Progressing	Documentation	Clinical notes Reflect related BH and medical conditions Useful to other team members	*30% of notes* *20% of team reports*	Offer training that addresses BH/medical comorbidities Standardized progress note-taking processes		
Progressing	Time management	Performs brief, targeted assessments and interventions Supports the clinic workflow	*45% of patients seen* *35% of team reports*	Offer training that addresses Patient engagement strategies Use of data from validated measures to inform work with patient BHP role and impact on clinic workflows		
Missing	Resource management	Refers patients to self-management resources and medical team supports	*0% of patients seen*	Offer training that addresses Identification of available resources that target BH issues		

References

American Psychological Association. (2015). *Competencies for psychology practice in primary care*. Retrieved from http://www.apa.org/ed/resources/competencies-practice.pdf.

American Psychological Association Education Directorate. (n.d.). *Directory of doctoral training programs with training opportunities in primary care psychology*. Retrieved from: http://www.apa.org/ed/graduate/primary-care-psychology.aspx

American Psychological Association, Interprofessional Seminar on Integrated Primary Care Work Group. (2016). *A curriculum for an interprofessional seminar on integrated primary care*. Retrieved from: http://www.apa.org/education/grad/curriculum-seminar.aspx

Baird, M., Hepworth, J., Myerholtz, L., & Reitz, R. (2017). Fifty years of contributions of behavioral science in family medicine. *Family Medicine, 49*(4), 296–303.

Blount, F. A., & Miller, B. F. (2009). Addressing the workforce crisis in integrated primary care. *Journal of Clinical Psychology in Medical Settings, 16*, 113–119.

Cubic, B., Mance, J., Turgesen, J. N., & Lamanna, J. D. (2012). Interprofessional education: Preparing psychologists for success in integrated care. *Journal of Clinical Psychology in Medical Settings, 19*, 84–92.

Curran, V., Heath, O., Adey, T., Callahan, T., Craig, D., Hearn, T., et al. (2012). An approach to integrating interprofessional education in collaborative mental health care. *Academic Psychiatry, 36*(2), 91–95.

Egnew, T. (2017). A philosophy for behavioral health integration in primary care. *Families, Systems & Health, 35*(1), 18–20.

Hall, J., Cohen, D. J., Davis, M., Gunn, R., Blount, A., Pollack, D. A., et al. (2015). Preparing the workforce for behavioral health and primary care integration. *Journal of the American Board of Family Medicine, 28*, S41–S51.

Hoge, M. A., Morris, J. A., Laraia, M., Pomerantz, A., & Farley, T. (2014). *Core competencies for integrated behavioral health and primary care*. Washington, DC: SAMHSA – HRSA Center for Integrated Health Solutions.

Institute for Healthcare Improvement (IHI). (2015). IHI Triple Aim Measures. Retrieved from http://www.ihi.org/engage/initiatives/TripleAim/Pages/MeasuresResults.aspx

Kinman, C., Gilchrist, E., Payne-Murphy, J., & Miller, B. (2015, March). *Provider- and practice-level competencies for integrated behavioral health in primary care: A literature review. (Prepared by Westat under Contract No. HHSA 290-2009-00023I)*. Rockville, MD: Agency for Healthcare Research and Quality.

Macchi, C.R. (2016, unpublished). *BHP performance evaluation tool.*

Macchi, C. R., Kessler, R., Auxier, A., Juvena, R., & Mullin, D. (2016). The practice integration profile: Rationale, development, method, and research. *Families, Systems & Health, 34*(4), 334–341.

Malott, K., Hall, K., Sheely-Moore, A., Krell, M., & Cardaciotto, L. (2014). Evidence-based teaching in higher education: Application to counselor education. *Counselor Education and Supervision, 53*, 294–305.

Martin, M. (2017). Integrated behavioral health training for primary care clinicians: Five lessons learned from a negative study. *Families, Systems, & Health*. ePub ahead of print.

Means, B., Toyama, Y., Murphy, R., Bakia, M., & Jones, K. (2009). *Evaluation of evidence-based practices in online learning: A meta-analysis and review of online learning studies*. Washington, DC: U.S. Department of Education, Office of Planning, Evaluation, and Policy Development.

Miller, B., Gilchrist, E., Ross, K., Wong, S. G., Blount, A., & Peek, C. J. (2016). *Core competencies for behavioral health providers working in primary care*. Retrieved from http://farleyhealthpolicycenter.org/wp-content/uploads/2016/02/Core-Competencies-for-Behavioral-Health-Providers-Working-in-Primary-Care.pdf

Peek, C. J. (2008). Planning care in the clinical, financial, and operational worlds. In R. Kessler & D. Stafford (Eds.), *Collaborative medicine case studies: Evidence in practice* (pp. 25–38). New York: Springer Science.

Reeves, S., Palaganas, J., & Zierler, B. (2017). An updated synthesis of review evidence of interprofessional education. *Journal of Allied Helath, 46*, 56–61.
Robinson, P. J., & Reiter, J. T. (2015). *Behavioral consultation and primary care: A guide to integrating services* (2nd ed.). Geneva, Switzerland: Springer International Publishing.
Serrano, N. (2015). *The implementer's guide to primary care behavioral health.* Madison, WI: Madison Community Health Centers.
Serrano, N., Cordes, C., Cubic, B., & Duab, S. (2017). The state and future of the primary care behavioral health workforce. *Journal of Clinical Psychology in Medical Settings.* ePub ahead of print.
Society for Health Psychology. (2018). Integrated primary care: An introductory curriculum. Retrieved from https://societyforhealthpsychology.org/training/integrated-primary-care-psychology/
Substance Abuse and Mental Health Services Administration-Health Resources and Services Administration Center for Integrated Care Solutions. (2014). *Advancing behavioral health integration within NCQA recognized patient-centered medical homes.* Retrieved from Washington, DC: https://www.integration.samhsa.gov/resource/advancing-behavioral-health-integration-within-ncqa-recognized-patient-centered-medical-homes
Wieman, C. (2014). Large-scale comparison of science teaching methods sends clear message. *Proceedings of the National Academy of Sciences, 111*(23), 8319–8320.

Chapter 10
Applied Data Analysis and Evaluation

Felicia Trembath and Stephanie Brennhofer

Chapter overview	
Domains	Data uses Develop a primary question and hypothesis Designing a research study Data collection Preparing data for statistical analysis Conducing the appropriate analysis
Key points	Statistical concepts should not be taught in isolation, but rather as a framework for health care professionals and administrators to think critically about health issues
Foundational knowledge and skills	Ability to recognize the appropriate types of studies to conduct in health care settings, basic knowledge of statistics, and recognition of the value of conducting studies in the health care setting
Student learning objectives (SLOs)	Upon completion of this chapter, the student will be able to: Formulate research questions and hypotheses Identify the key issues commonly encountered with biomedical data Know which key issues to be aware of, based on data usage Know how to prevent these issues from influencing the accuracy of their results or interpretations Explain the procedures for cleaning data Identify proper statistical methods based on the hypotheses of a study Interpret statistical results to determine statistical and clinical significance
Instructional strategies	Provide mock datasets and examples to guide learners through the steps of developing a research question, designing a study, collecting data, preparing data, conducting the proper statistical analysis, and interpreting the results
Evaluating learning	Identify the steps to conducting a study Go through each step in conducting a study using a mock data set

F. Trembath (✉) · S. Brennhofer
Integrated Behavioral Health Programs, College of Health Solutions,
Arizona State University, Phoenix, AZ, USA
e-mail: ftrembat@asu.edu; Stephanie.Brennhofer@asu.edu

C. R. Macchi, R. Kessler (eds.), *Training to Deliver Integrated Care*,
https://doi.org/10.1007/978-3-319-78850-0_10

Historical Approaches to Statistical Training

This chapter provides statistical teaching strategies for trainers who provide instruction and direction to practicing professionals. In academic settings, students are taught the basic concepts of statistics, specific statistical techniques, and statistical tests that may be conducted. However, the examples and datasets employed in academic settings are often devoid of the issues that may be encountered when working with real data in the workplace. As such, practicing health care professionals may understand statistical concepts and how to run specific tests, but lack an understanding of how to avoid and deal with the key issues prevalent in collecting, analyzing, and interpreting biomedical data. This chapter aims to tackle those issues while providing insight on how a trainer can teach these statistical concepts to clinicians and health care administrators by discussing common uses for health care data, how to formulate a hypothesis and propose a data inquiry or "study," types of study designs, key statistical issues, and the steps to prepare the data for analysis, such as understanding assumptions of statistical tests, conducting the appropriate analysis, and interpreting the results. Each topic will include real-world examples that engage trainers and trainees in applied analysis in practice settings.

Common Data Uses

Although there are many possible uses for biomedical data, the most common uses of data in medical settings are (1) conducting program or clinical evaluations and (2) using data from existing sources, such as electronic health records (EHRs). A potential program evaluation could examine the effectiveness of a clinic that provides high-need patients with transportation to reduce the number of missed appointments. An example of using EHR data could be illustrated when a clinician or administrator explores the associations of HbA1C levels and the types of patient health insurance plans.

Conducting Evaluation As we move toward a more intense data analytic environment, we need more health care professionals and administrators who can work with the data provided in their health care setting. The current health care climate reflects an increased focus on demonstrating improvements in patient outcomes. Reimbursements may be tied to the ability to demonstrate these improvements. Addressing the associations between outcomes and reimbursements requires health care centers to collect and analyze data that facilitate conducting treatment and program evaluations. Trainers will need to train clinicians and health care administrators on the statistical issues to be aware of and to be considered in the design and execution of a program or treatment evaluation. It is imperative when collecting data for a program evaluation that the information needing to be collected is thought out beforehand.

Using Existing Data As a trainer, it is essential that your clinicians and health care administrators understand the information that is available to them via the EHR and how that data can be used in a reasonable way to inform practices and improve clinical outcomes. Given the vast array of data available through the EHR, it is tempting to dive right into the data. However, this practice increases the chance of finding an erroneous result. In order to avoid this, this chapter will serve as a guide on the most important items for a trainer to teach health care professionals and administrators. Such training will help ensure that reliable analyses are being conducted to inform clinical practices and programmatic decisions.

Key Conceptual and Operational Shifts in Statistical Training

As the health care system has changed, so has the need for clinicians and administrators to learn how to perform basic statistical analyses. We are past the days where statistics are only to be conducted by statisticians or researchers in academic settings. Table 10.1 shows the shift that should and is occurring with the use of statistics.

The following sections provide a process-oriented approach for trainers to lead learners through a series of steps starting with a main research question and ending with an answer to that question. All major sections are labeled as "steps" that occur in a sequential order to effectively train clinicians and administrators to perform applied statistics within health care settings. Key statistical issues to be aware of at each step are identified and discussed.

Step 1: Develop a Primary Question and Hypotheses

Before diving into the data, it is important for clinicians and administrators to think about what they are interested in and why. To start with, a primary research question, which is the broad question that an individual hopes to answer, needs to be

Table 10.1 Change in statistical use over time

Academic Setting	Health Care Setting
Theoretical or application-based	Application-based
Traditional statistics training • A required class for select undergraduate majors (e.g., psychology majors) focused on the mechanics of performing statistical analyses • Required coursework for graduate students to perform research • To prepare future statisticians	Workforce development addressing applied statistics in health care settings • Clinicians and administrators perform basic statistical analyses with health care center data • Evaluate program effectiveness, clinical outcomes, and health care delivery costs

formulated. Each research question will generally have several hypotheses, which are logical assumptions that are based on prior research or known facts and that can be tested. The distinction between a research question and hypothesis may not be readily apparent to the trainees. The main difference between the two is that a research question states a general area of interest, while the hypothesis translates the research question into a form that can be tested. When formulating the hypothesis, trainees should begin to think about what they want to examine. For example, do they want to examine the relationship between two variables or do they want to examine differences between groups? To illustrate the difference between a research question and a hypothesis, here are some examples of research questions and the resulting hypotheses for each of the two most common data use examples mentioned above:

Program Evaluation Primary Question: Does implementing a transportation program for high-need patients reduce the number of missed appointments?

Hypothesis: Engagement in the transportation program will decrease the number of missed appointments by 50% within the first 3 months.

Existing Data Primary Question: Among patients with diabetes, is there a relationship between the type of health insurance that a patient has and their HbA1C level?

Hypothesis 1: Patients with diabetes who are without health insurance will have higher HbA1C levels than patients with diabetes who have health insurance.

Hypothesis 2: Patients with diabetes who have a high-deductible health plan or health saving accounts (HSA) will have higher HbA1C levels than patients with diabetes who have a preferred provider organization (PPO) or exclusive provider organization (EPO) for health insurance.

Hypothesis 3: Patients with diabetes who have a health maintenance organization (HMO) health plan will have higher HbA1C levels than patients with diabetes who have a PPO or EPO.

It is critical that trainers communicate the importance of formulating proper primary research questions and hypotheses as they will be the driving force of the statistical inquiry. In order to do this, trainees must begin to think about the definitions they are going to use to form their hypotheses. For example, a clinician may begin with a very broad question such as are group counseling sessions for patients with depression successful? They have to be guided to think through how success will be defined. Will it be based on the patient's score on an assessment tool? If so, which assessment tool will be utilized? Usually there are multiple ways that something can be defined, and rather than focusing on getting the "correct" answer, it is more important that trainees begin to think about how to establish definitions in order to translate their research question into a testable hypothesis. The main statistical issue to be aware of during step 1 is fishing.

Fishing Fishing is the term used when an individual explores a dataset by running preliminary statistics for interesting and/or statistically significant results without determining a hypothesis a priori (i.e., before the fact). In other words, they are searching for a result that they like. Fishing is an issue, because it violates the scientific assumptions of hypothesis testing and makes it more likely that a statistically significant result will be found due to chance alone.

The trainees must understand the difference between developing a hypothesis and then conducting the statistical analysis versus fishing in the dataset for a result that is significant by running multiple statistical tests. If clinicians are using an existing dataset, they may look at the dataset to see what variables are present and in what measurement scale the information was collected. This knowledge will guide their hypothesis development and test selection. However, the statistical analysis should not be completed without a specific hypothesis that will be tested using that dataset.

During step 1, trainers can find out what their trainees are most passionate about in regard to health care data collection and program evaluation. By finding out the passions of those you train, you can use examples that they are interested in to guide them down the route of research question and hypothesis formation. The importance of step 1 cannot be overstated, as a well-founded hypothesis is the underpinning of conducting a proper statistical analysis.

Step 2: Design the Study

Some clinicians and administrators may be interested in designing and conducting their own study. Perhaps they have a question they would like to answer, but the health care center is not currently collecting the requisite data. In this instance, the individual will need to think about how they would like to go about collecting this information. Proper consideration in the design phase is essential. When training clinicians and administrators on how to properly design a study, they need to be guided to think though: (1) exactly what research question they want to answer; (2) what information needs to be collected in order to answer that question; (3) any issues, including potential confounders, that need to be considered; (4) what study designs could be used to answer this question; (5) the measurement scale for data collection; (6) the appropriate statistical test to address their hypothesis; and (7) the level of significance that they will set for their study. During the design phase, clinicians must be aware of the statistical issues of measurement scale, confounders, type I and type II error, clustered data, establishing cause and effect, test selection, and generalizability.

Measurement Scale The method of measuring a variable will vary based on what information is being collected. For example, speed at performing a task may be measured with a stopwatch, while patient reported pain level will likely be measured using a Likert-type scale with options ranging from 1 to 10. Measurement scales can be described as nominal, ordinal, or interval/ratio; see Table 10.2 for a description and examples of each.

When dealing with existing data, researchers are constrained to how the variables have already been collected. On the other hand, when researchers are collecting data, they must decide how the variables of interest will be measured and collected. For example, if age is a variable of interest, will it be collected as an open field ranging from 0 to 99, or will age groups be divided into categories, such as 0–19, 20–39, 40–59, and 60–99? Nonnumerical data cannot be analyzed in the same way that numerical data can be, thus, different statistical tests are appropriate for different measurement scales. During the design phase, trainees should be guided to consider what statistical tests are appropriate for the measurement scale that they will be using.

Confounders A confounder is a variable that is associated with both the exposure and the outcome (see Fig. 10.1); if not taken into consideration, confounders may distort the relationship between the exposure and the outcome.

For example, there is an association between alcohol consumption and heart disease. However, cigarette smoking is a behavior that is related to both alcohol

Table 10.2 Measurement scales

Measurement scale	Description	Examples
Nominal	Used for labeling variables that do not have quantitative value	Gender, religious preference, presence of diabetes (yes or no)
Ordinal	Characteristics that can be rank ordered, but the distance between the values does not have inherent meaning	Pain scales, patient satisfaction
Interval/ratio	Numerical values where the distance between each value does have meaning	Weight, age, HbA1C levels

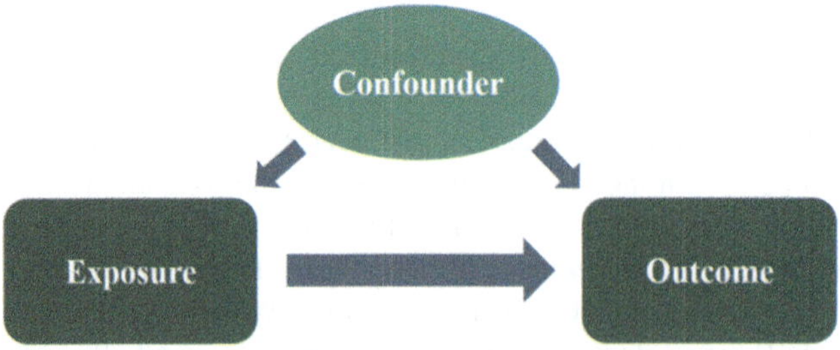

Fig. 10.1 The relationship of confounders

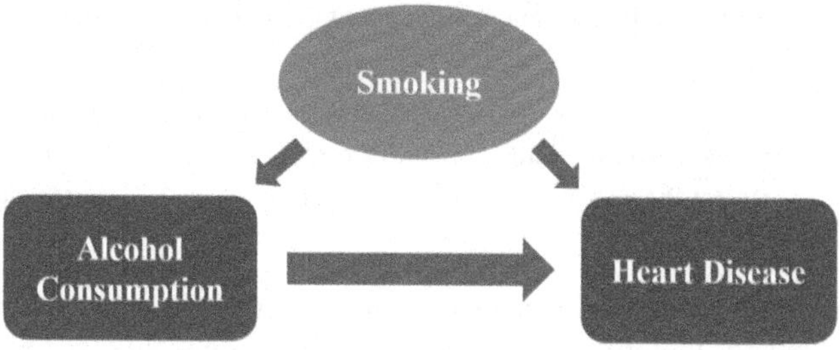

Fig. 10.2 The relationship of confounders: smoking example

consumption and heart disease. If a study examining the relationship between alcohol consumption and heart disease fails to consider whether participants smoke cigarettes, the true relationship between alcohol consumption and heart disease may be distorted (see Fig. 10.2). During the design phase, researchers should think about potential confounders, and develop a plan to collect information on them. For example, if smoking is a potential confounder, then researchers should develop a plan to collect information on smoking habits. Depending upon the type of statistical analysis chosen, confounders may be controlled for by including them in the statistical model.

Type I and Type II Error In hypothesis testing, the null hypothesis states there is no effect, while the alternative hypothesis is phrased to test the effect of interest. In the practice of medicine, there are no absolutes; similarly with statistics we never know the truth for certain. Instead we are dealing with probabilities and making our decision about whether or not to reject the null hypothesis based on the results of statistical tests. Basically, a threshold is set indicating at what point the results would likely not be due to chance, but rather due to the variable that is being measured. This can be done by one of two methods (1) comparing the calculated test statistic value to the critical value for the chosen test or (2) by comparing the *p*-value to the significance level chosen by the researcher during the design phase of the study. The *p*-value represents the probability of getting the given statistical result if the null hypothesis is true. Since the *p*-value is a probability, it will always be a value between zero and one. The *p*-value method is used most commonly in practice to determine statistical significance, because it is frequently provided with the output from statistical tests and is always in the same scale, thus making it easier to interpret across different statistical methods. During the design phase of the study, the researcher will choose the level of significance to be used. In theory any value between 0 and 1 can be chosen, however, in practice researchers will typically choose either 0.10, 0.05, or 0.01. The most commonly used significance level is 0.05, although researchers may want to use a lower significance level when they want to be more certain that they would not conclude the results are statistically significant when in fact the null hypothesis is true. For example, when dealing with medical decisions, we would want to be as certain as possible that the statistical results are valid before changing treatment protocols. In this case, a researcher may

Table 10.3 How reality and the decision made can lead to a correct conclusion or error

		Reality	
		Null is true	**Null is false**
Decision	**Fail to reject the null**	Correct decision	Type II error
	Reject the null	Type I error	Correct decision

chose the more stringent significance level of 0.01. A *p*-value that is lower than the level of significance that was set during the design phase would lead the researcher to conclude that the given statistical result is very unlikely to be due to chance and thus that the null hypothesis should be rejected. The null hypothesis assumes that there is no effect. When the null hypothesis is rejected, the researcher is concluding that the result is statistically significant. Because statistics deal with probabilities, there is always the possibility that the decision made is wrong. Table 10.3 illustrates the relationship between the reality of a situation and the decision that is made to reject or fail to reject the null hypothesis.

As we see in Table 10.3, a type I error occurs when the null hypothesis is rejected when it is actually true, while a type II error occurs when the null hypothesis is not rejected when it is actually false. Typically 0.05 is chosen as the significance level, because it is thought of as the level that best balances the possibility of making a correct decision with the possibility of committing a type I or type II error. If 0.05 is chosen as the significance level, a statistical result with $p < 0.05$ would be considered statistically significant. Since the *p*-value reflects the probability of getting the statistical result that you got if the null hypothesis is in fact true, a *p*-value of 0.05 indicates there is a 5% chance of getting the given result from the statistical test if the null hypothesis is in fact true. A lower *p*-value, for example, 0.01, would indicate that it is even more unlikely that the results are by chance. However, even with a small *p*-value, it is possible that the null hypothesis is true and there actually is no difference. Every time a statistical test is run, there is a chance of making the wrong decision and committing a type I or type II error. Thus, it is important for trainers to caution their trainees on running multiple tests. Recall the discussion from step 1 on fishing for a result in the dataset; running numerous analyses in an effort to find a significant result increases the likelihood that an error will be committed and that a statistical result would be found by chance alone. This phenomenon is referred to as alpha inflation.

Clustered Data Clustered data occurs when the data from a dataset can be divided into different groups (i.e., clusters). A cluster could be the patients from each doctor, a family unit, or an individual patient with multiple observations. Conceptually, the data points within each cluster are likely to be more similar to each other than to other observations in the dataset. With practice-based biomedical data, clustered data most frequently occurs when there are multiple observations per person in the same dataset (e.g., multiple diagnostic codes per visit, multiple gestation pregnancies, or multiple pregnancies within the observed time period). Conceptually, the multiple observations from an individual person are probably more like the observations from that same person than to the observations from an unrelated person in the database, which could violate the assumption of independence and create some challenges to data analysis. Failure to consider the clustered nature of data could lead to results that are not accurate or a study that lacks sufficient power to find an effect. Specialized data techniques can be used to analyze the data. These techniques require advanced training or statistical consultation, which should be considered when there are serious concerns about clustered data. A simpler technique that could be employed would be to limit the analysis to one observation per person. For example, if a clinician or administrator has a database with labor and delivery information that spans a 5-year period, it is likely that some of the women in the database will have had multiple deliveries during that time; the simplest way to deal with this issue would be to analyze only the first pregnancy from each woman. This means that second and subsequent pregnancies that occur in the database would be excluded from the analysis. Although there are some limitations to this approach, it is feasible to accomplish and is a better strategy than ignoring the fact that the data is clustered.

Establishing Cause and Effect In biomedical studies, it may not be enough to show that two variables are related to each other; we frequently want to establish cause and effect. The gold standard study design for determining cause and effect is a randomized controlled trial (RCT) where participants are selected and then randomized to a treatment group or control group. However, when evaluating medical research questions, RCTs are not always feasible or ethically possible. For example, researchers evaluating the effect of a medication during pregnancy cannot randomize women to either be pregnant or not be pregnant. Additionally, there has been a recent shift from clinical trials to pragmatic trials (Ford & Norrie, 2016). The shift occurred given the discrepancy that is sometimes seen between what is conducted in a controlled research environment versus what actually occurs in clinical practice. Common study designs used in biomedical research to evaluate causation are shown in Table 10.4.

Test Selection When deciding which statistical test is appropriate to conduct, trainees should consider the measurement scale of the variables as well as what they want to examine. Not all statistical tests are appropriate for different types of data. For example, a mean cannot be calculated for nominal level data, since nominal data is dividing participants based on attributes, such as gender, and has no intrinsic numerical value. Additionally, it is not uncommon for researchers to analyze ordinal level data as though it was interval/ratio, an example being reporting a mean and standard deviation for patient satisfaction ratings that are scored on a five-point Likert-type scale. Results like these should be interpreted with caution, since ordinal level data does not have intrinsic numerical values and is often measuring subjective attitudes. For example, on a five-point Likert-type scale, the distance between a four (satisfied) and a five (very satisfied) is not necessarily going to be the same for every patient. Statistical tests appropriate to the measurement scale should be selected. The decision about which test is appropriate will also be influenced by what a person wants to examine. For example, does the trainee want to look at the relationship between two variables, such as the relationship between age and sys-

Table 10.4 Types of study designs

Study design	Description	Type of study
Cohort	A group of people (cohort) is selected and either analyzed prospectively or retrospectively to evaluate the risk factors associated with the outcome of interest	Observational
Case-control	Persons with the outcome of interest (cases) and persons who are similar but without the outcome of interest (controls) are selected. Information is analyzed to evaluate the risk factors associated with the outcome of interest	Observational
Randomized controlled trial	Participants are selected and randomly assigned to a treatment or control group	Experimental

tolic blood pressure, or do they want to look at differences between groups, such as the difference in HbA1C levels based on treatment protocol. It is important that the statistical test to be utilized is considered during the design phase, in order to ensure that the proper data is collected and proper procedures are followed. There are myriad statistical techniques for dealing with the varying situations that might occur when conducting research. An in-depth discussion of these tests is beyond the scope of this training manual. However, a decision tree depicting the most common statistical tests based on measurement scale of the dependent variable is presented in Fig. 10.3.

Generalizability Generalizability refers to the ability to extrapolate findings beyond the sample studied to the entire population of interest. There is no statistical test to determine generalizability; rather it is a decision made by those evaluating the results based on the factors prevalent in the study. When evaluating generalizability, there are several factors that should be considered, including sample selection and sample size.

Sample Selection In order for findings to be generalizable, the sample that a clinician or administrator chooses to use needs to be a representative of the population of interest and an adequate size. Having a representative sample means that the demographics (e.g., age, race/ethnicity, gender) of the study sample should mirror that of the population of interest. For example, if the health care center has patients with an average age of 25 and is comprised of 40% Hispanic individuals, the sample selected should also have an average age close to 25 and should be comprised of approximately 40% Hispanic individuals to be able to effectively extrapolate their findings to their entire clinic. However, it is not always possible to get a sample that is directly representative of the population being examined. In cases such as these, it is imperative that the narrative is reworded to what the findings from an inquiry can actually say about a population. For example, if the clinic in the above example was only able to get data on predominantly non-Hispanic patients, then their findings would extrapolate to the non-Hispanic individuals in their clinic, not the entire clinic.

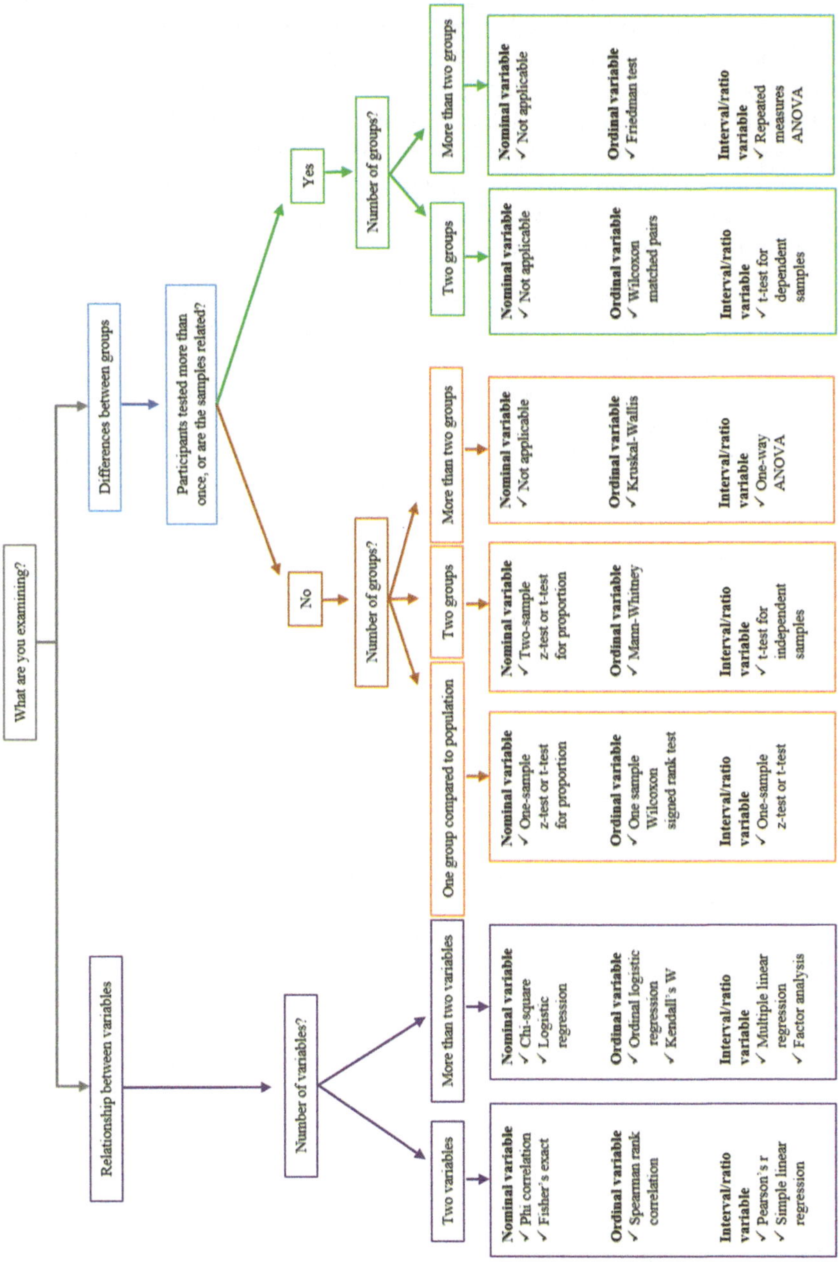

Fig. 10.3 Decision tree for choosing a statistical test

Another very important point for trainees to understand is that the sample selected for the study should have been selected in a way that each member of the population had an equal chance of being selected. A study will be doomed before it begins if the sample is somehow "stacked" in a way that nearly guarantees a desired result. For example, if a trainee would like to evaluate the effectiveness of a new diabetes management program, but specifically targets those who have made the most improvement throughout the program and neglects to equally include those who have made little or no improvement, the study is biased in such a manner that the results are void of any merit. As tempting as it may be for trainees to select out their most compliant or nicest patients, this introduces significant bias and will undermine the results of the study.

Sample Size The larger the sample size, the better the estimate of the true population parameter. Sample size highly influences the ability of a study to demonstrate a statistically significant effect, especially the ability to detect small differences between groups. The ability to detect an effect, if one is actually present, is referred to as power. Often researchers evaluate power as a post hoc test (i.e., after the fact) to explain nonsignificant results. However, the sample size needed to have adequate power can, and should, be calculated during the design phase of a study. When calculating sample size, the known information about the condition being studied and the chosen statistical parameters (e.g., the prevalence of the outcome and the desired significance level) are used to compute the necessary sample size. The formula for determining sample size will vary based on the type of study being conducted. Some statistical programs have functions to calculate sample size, but there is also a plethora of online sample size calculators.

Step 3: Data Acquisition

Once the elements of the study design have been properly thought out, the next step is to acquire the data. In the study design phase, the trainees were guided to develop a list of all variables that would be required to test their hypothesis; this list will guide the data acquisition process. Depending upon the hypothesis being tested, data acquisition may be through primary data collection or by obtaining access to previously collected data.

Prior to beginning any data collection, a method to house the data must be developed, which could be something relatively simple such as an Excel file or something more complicated such as a customized database. The process for getting data into the database must also be determined. In some cases it may be possible to set up a database with fields that auto-populate based on information from the patient's EHR, however, in most situations some manual data entry will be required. Several procedures should be put in place to ensure that quality data will be collected. First, a standardized format for data entry should be established. Decisions to make include how variables will be recorded (e.g., will weight be recorded in pounds or

Table 10.5 Sample codebook

Variable name	Explanation	Format	Example
Patient ID	Unique study identification number for each patient	6 digit number	123456
Weight	Patient's weight in kilograms	2–5 digit number	68.05
Last visit	The date of the patient's last visit	8 digit number	02/04/2015
Physician	Last name of the patient's treating physician	All capital letters	SMITH

kilograms) and whether or not words will be capitalized. If proper thought is not put into the database development, there will likely be numerous issues when preparing the data for analysis. For example, if patient weight is being collected and sometimes weight is recorded in pounds while other times it is recorded in kilograms, this must be corrected by the researcher before any analysis can be conducted. From a statistical analysis standpoint, it does not matter whether weight is recorded in pounds or kilograms; what does matter is that the data entry format is consistent. Second, a codebook explaining each variable should be developed. The codebook serves as a reference when several people alternate doing data entry and also serves as reference for the researcher when the database is reviewed at a later time period. The term codebook sounds formal but simply refers to a table or list with the definition of each variable and the format for how it should be entered. The codebook can be kept as a separate file or as an additional page or tab in the database. A sample data codebook is represented in Table 10.5.

If an existing dataset is to be utilized for analysis, the researcher must gain access to the data. The method of procurement will vary based on the data being utilized. For example, if a clinician wants to extract information from an organization's existing EHR, they will need to identify and work with a person in the organization who can mine the EHR system in order to download the requisite information. Even if existing data is being used, a method of housing the data still needs to be developed, and a codebook should be created to serve as a reference point.

Step 4: Prepare the Data for Analysis

Once data has been collected, it needs to be cleaned (i.e., prepared) for analysis. During this step the data is reviewed in order to make sure that it makes sense and is free from errors. An easy way to check the data for errors is through conducting simple frequency analyses and to graph the data as a histogram. It is important to visualize the data as problems may not be apparent by looking at numbers alone. Datasets drawn from real-life data can be messy and take a substantial amount of cleaning; the main issues to be aware of are missing information, outliers, generalizability, and statistical assumptions.

Missing Information When working with biomedical data, missing information is a common issue. Consider a physician who wishes to track the blood glucose levels of their patients in order to evaluate the impact of a new diabetes behavioral intervention. This may sound like a simple idea and process, however, there are several intervening steps to get the blood glucose values into the data management software. First, a database must be created to house the data. Second, the physician must order the lab work. Third, unless the bloodwork can be done in the physician's office at the same time as the appointment, the patient must go to a lab to have the blood drawn. Fourth, the results of the bloodwork must be either automatically populated or manually added to the database. Fifth, other important information (e.g., height, weight, age) must be manually added to database. Any one of these points can break down, resulting in missing information. Great care should be taken to complete the missing information. This could necessitate reviewing patient records, contacting the laboratory for results, or following up with the patient directly. In a database of any substantial size, this process can be very time-consuming. However, it is of paramount importance to complete as much of the missing information as possible, in order to maintain the integrity of the data. If missing information cannot be located, this must be taken into account in the data analysis. The exact procedures will vary depending on the software being used, but a coding scheme that indicates which values are missing should be applied.

Outliers An outlier is an extreme data point that is far outside the expected range of values. Because these values are so disparate from the rest of the distribution, outliers can affect the mean and create skewness in the dataset, which could cause some errors in data analysis and interpretation. Outliers can be detected by computing frequency tables and by graphing the data using histograms or boxplots. There are differing opinions on the best way to handle outliers. In order to have a clean dataset, trainees may be tempted to remove outliers, however, this is not necessarily the best course of action. When an outlier is detected, further review is warranted to try to determine the cause. An outlier may indicate that some sort of error has occurred. For example, with survey data, maybe the patient did not understand the question that was being asked, or maybe the person doing the data entry accidentally typed in the wrong value. If an outlier is suspected to be an erroneous value, efforts should be taken to verify the accuracy of the value by reviewing original records where available. On the other hand, an extreme value could be a legitimate result that represents variation in the population. For example, if a researcher is collecting height information for individuals, some people may be very short, while others may be very tall. If it can be concluded with reasonable certainty that the outlier is due to some sort of error which cannot be corrected, it can be removed from the dataset. However, if the outlier could be a legitimate result due to natural variation in the population or some other factor, it should be left as is, even if this necessitates more complicated data analysis techniques. Trainees should be able to articulate whether there are outliers, what they are going to do with the outliers, and the rationale for their actions.

As discussed in step 3, the necessity for data cleaning due to data entry issues can be minimized by establishing the database prior to beginning data collection, establishing a standardized format for data entry, and keeping a codebook that explains each variable.

Generalizability Although generalizability was considered in the study design phase, it must also be considered once the data has actually been collected. During step 4, the data will be checked to ensure that the procedures for generalizability developed during the study design phase have been followed. Specifically trainees will ensure that the final sample is representative of the population of interest, that the sample was collected in such a way that every member of the population of interest was equally likely to be chosen, and that the final sample size is adequate to address the hypothesis.

Statistical Assumptions Every statistical test is based on background assumptions about the data being analyzed. It is important that the trainees understand all the fundamental assumptions of the statistical test that they choose to use. One of the basic assumptions underlying many statistical tests is that the data is normally distributed, which is represented by a bell-shaped curve (see Fig. 10.4). In a normal distribution it is known what percentage of observations will fall in each portion of the curve, with the majority of the observations clustered around the mean, and 68% of observations falling within ±1 standard deviation from the mean.

It is important that trainees understand that biomedical data may not follow a perfectly normal distribution, particularly if a subgroup is being examined. For example, if evaluating systolic blood pressure measurements for a random sample of patients, the results would likely follow a normal distribution. However, if a clinic is interested in knowing whether or not a behavioral intervention is effective at reducing systolic blood pressure measurements for hypertensive patients, the systolic blood pressure measurements for these patients will likely be higher than for the general population, and may not follow a normal distribution. Smaller datasets (particularly ones with fewer than 30 observations) are more prone to having an abnormal distribution, since outliers will have a more profound effect on the distribution of the data as a whole. On the other hand, when dealing with larger datasets, there are often enough data points to counterbalance a few outliers, which means that as a whole the data will have a normal distribution.

If the statistical test being utilized assumes that the data is normally distributed, the normality of the dataset needs to be ascertained before the statistical test is run. There are some formal tests that can be utilized to assess the normality of a distribution; however, each of these has limitations. A practical approach to assessing normality is to evaluate the skewness and kurtosis of the distribution.

Skewness Skewness refers to the asymmetry of a distribution. In a normal distribution, the distribution is perfectly symmetric and if folded in half would perfectly match. Outliers on either the lower or upper ends of the distribution can result in a skewed distribution. In a positively skewed distribution, the tail points toward the

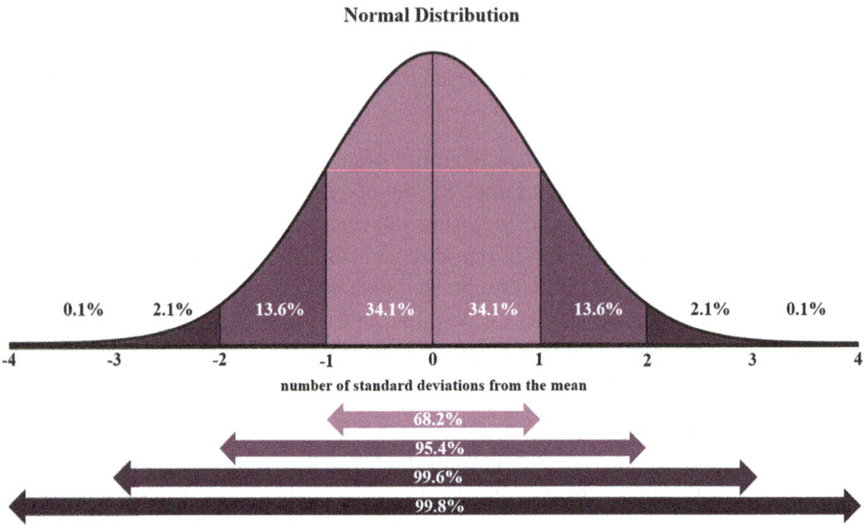

Fig. 10.4 Normal distribution curve

positive values, while in a negatively skewed distribution, the tail points toward the negative values (see Fig. 10.5). Skewness can be calculated separately but is typically part of the results provided in the output from the descriptive statistics function. The skew of a normal distribution will be equal to zero. Although there are differing viewpoints on the cutoff point for determining skewness, a rule of thumb is that a skew of more than ±2 is problematic, and the data cannot be assumed to be normally distributed (George & Mallery, 2010).

Kurtosis There are differing opinions on exactly what kurtosis represents. Historically, kurtosis has been described as the measure of the peakedness of a distribution, however, some modern statisticians contend that instead kurtosis is actually measuring the weight of the tails of the distribution (Westfall, 2014). Regardless of the way that it is conceptualized, what kurtosis is describing is the dispersion of the observations in a distribution, and whether or not they conform to the pattern expected within a normal distribution. Recall that in a normal distribution it is known what percentage of observations will fall under each portion of the curve, as depicted in Fig. 10.4. If the data in a given sample does not follow a normal distribution but instead has either a higher or lower percentage of the observations in the tails, this could lead the researcher to make erroneous statistical conclusions. Mathematically the kurtosis of a normal distribution is equal to three. A distribution with positive kurtosis has fewer observations around the mean, and more outliers. This results in a distribution with a narrower peak and fatter tails. On the other hand, a distribution with negative kurtosis has more observations that are a moderate distance from the mean, and few outliers. This results in a rounded or mound-shaped distribution (see Fig. 10.6). Some statistical software, such as Excel and SPSS, evaluate the excess kurtosis, which in effect assigns a kurtosis of zero to a normal

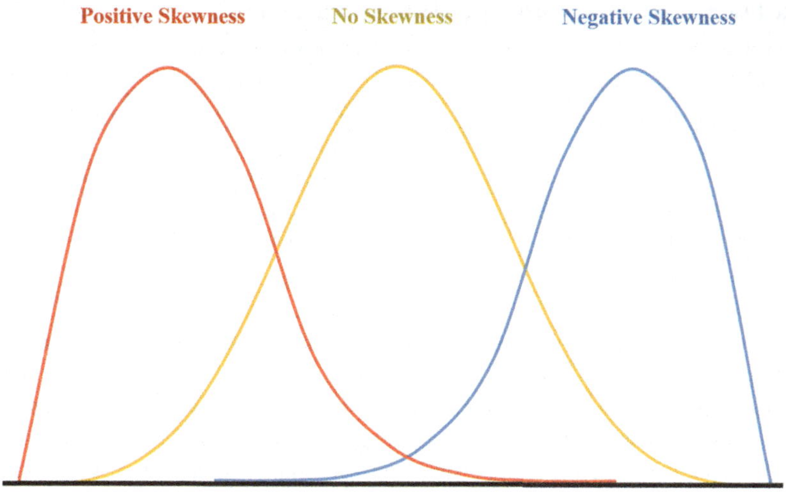

Fig. 10.5 Types of skewness

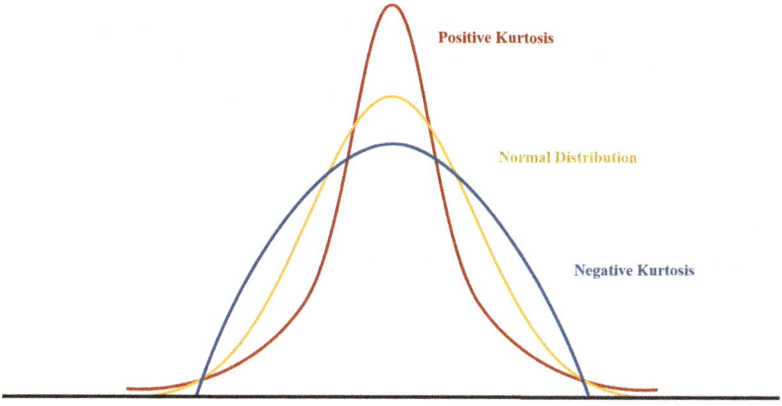

Fig. 10.6 Types of kurtosis

distribution. When evaluating kurtosis, it is essential to know what method the statistical software being employed uses. Kurtosis can be calculated separately but is typically part of the results provided in the output from the descriptive statistics function. A good rule of thumb is that kurtosis more than ±2 from the expected value is considered substantial, and the data cannot be assumed to be normally distributed (George & Mallery, 2010).

In the design phase, trainees have already thought through what statistical tests would be appropriate to use based on what measurement scale the variables collected are in and what they want to evaluate. If the statistical assumptions for the test

Table 10.6 Parametric tests and the equivalent nonparametric tests

Parametric tests	Nonparametric tests
t-test for independent samples	Mann-Whitney test
t-test for dependent samples	Wilcoxon matched-pairs signed rank test
ANOVA	Kruskal-Wallis test
Pearson correlation	Spearman rank-order correlation
Linear regression	Nonparametric regression
Two-sample proportions test	Chi-square

that they chose to use are violated, additional work with the data will be required, or a different statistical method will need to be selected. How this situation will be handled depends on which statistical assumption has been violated. In terms of the assumption of a normal distribution, statistical tests are classified as either parametric or nonparametric. Parametric tests assume normality of the data, while nonparametric tests do not. If the data is not normally distributed, clinicians and administrators have several options, including using the parametric test anyway, mathematically transforming the data, or choosing an equivalent nonparametric test. Both determining whether or not a sample size is large enough for a parametric test to be valid and mathematically transforming the data may require some advanced statistical training that practicing professionals may not have received. As a practical matter, if the data is not normally distributed, a nonparametric test appropriate to the research question should be selected. Table 10.6 contains a list of common parametric tests and the nonparametric counterpart.

Step 5: Conduct the Appropriate Analysis

Once the data has been prepared for analysis and the statistical assumptions underlying the chosen test have been checked to ensure that they are met, the next step is to conduct the analysis and make conclusions based on the results. When making conclusions, a key issue to be aware of is the difference between statistical and clinical significance.

Statistical Significance Versus Clinical Significance Statistical significance is concerned with whether or not a result is a valid result, meaning it is unlikely to have occured by chance. A conclusion about whether or not a test is statistically significant is made either (1) by comparing the calculated test statistic to the critical value for the chosen test or (2) by comparing the obtained p-value to the significance level set during the design phase. As discussed previously, comparing the p-value to the significance level is the method most commonly used in practice. If a result is determined to be statistically significant, we must then consider the clinical (also called practical) significance, which addresses whether or not results are relevant in the real world. There are some statistics that can aid in the interpretation of clinical significance, such as a measure of effect. A measure of effect (also called effect size) is a statistic that measures the magnitude of the relationship or difference that is seen. There are various measures of effect for different statistical tests, including odds ratio, relative risk, Cohen's d, correlation, and variance. Since measures of effect quantify the magnitude of an effect, they can aid in determining whether a result has clinical significance. However, trainees should understand that clinical significance is a matter of judgment, based on the findings of the research study and the expertise of practitioners. It is imperative that trainers keep the concept of clinical significance in mind while training clinicians and administrators to analyze data. When evaluating a statistically significant finding, it is important to ask, "Is this clinically relevant?". For example, a clinic may want to evaluate the effectiveness of a new weight loss program they implemented 6 months ago. Upon statistical analysis, they found that on average people lost 0.5 pounds, which was statistically significant as evidenced by a *p*-value <0.05. It is at this point that clinicians and administrators need to ask themselves if losing half a pound over the course of 6 months is clinically relevant. One way to conceptualize clinical significance is for clinicians to ask themselves whether or not the finding is meaningful enough for them to alter their practice. In summary, statistical significance deals with the likelihood that a result is authentic, while clinical significance is a subjective interpretation of the meaningfulness of the results. Through training exercises, clinicians and administrators should be taught to understand the difference between statistical and clinical significance and be encouraged to always think through and justify why they believe that a statistically significant result is or is not clinically significant.

Measurement of Effective Statistical Training

While there are many ways to gauge the effectiveness of statistical training, perhaps the simplest and least intimidating way is through a mock dataset. As the trainer, you will provide this dataset, and based on the information available, trainees need to develop research questions and hypotheses, design the study, prepare the data for analysis, run the analysis, and make a decision about the statistical and clinical significance of the results. For advanced trainees, they may have a dataset that they are already working with that they can use during the course. The five steps to conducting a study that will be taught during the course can be broken down into individual training sessions covering the key concepts.

The following checklist can serve as a guide for each trainee during each of the five steps to ensure that each step is fully completed (see Table 10.7). The chart needs to be followed in numerical order of each step. When filling out the chart below for each trainee, if an answer is "no," the trainee needs to be stopped and must make the necessary changes until the answer to the item is "yes." They are not to proceed onto the next step until the prior step is filled with "yes" answers, or they can provide sufficient justification for a "no" answer.

Table 10.7 Sample evaluation template

Steps and sub-steps	Items	Yes/No
Step 1: Develop a primary question and hypotheses		
Research question	Broad question was identified	
Definitions	Can articulate relevant definitions (i.e., how improvement is defined)	
Hypothesis	It is logical	
	It can be tested	
	It can be measured	
	It is based on prior research or known facts	
Fishing	Can articulate the issues created by fishing	
	Dataset was not explored prior to research question and hypothesis formation	
Step 2: Design the study		
Study design	Will address hypotheses	
	Is feasible	
	Resources are available to conduct	
Requisite variables	Can identify variables needed to address hypothesis	
Confounders	Can identify potential confounders that need to be considered	
Measurement scale	Can identify what type of variables will be collected	
Type I and type II error	Can articulate what a type I error would mean for their dataset	
	Can articulate what a type II error would mean for their dataset	
	A reasonable number of tests are proposed to avoid alpha inflation	
Clustered data	Potential clustering of data was considered	
Generalizability	Participant selection is random and will likely result in representative sample	
	Consideration has been given to the requisite sample size	
	If relevant, sample size calculation has been performed	
Test selection	Selected statistical test is appropriate for the hypothesis and measurement scale	
	Can articulate the assumptions of chosen statistical test	
Step 3: Data collection		
Data acquisition	If relevant, point of contact for obtaining data has been identified	
Data management	Database for data management has been developed	
	Standardized data entry format has been developed	
	Codebook has been established	
Step 4: Prepare the data for analysis		
Missing information	Data was evaluated for missing information	
	A method was developed to deal with missing information	

(continued)

Table 10.7 (continued)

Steps and sub-steps	Items	Yes/No
Outliers	Data was graphed to check for outliers	
	Can articulate the need to remove or keep each outlier in dataset	
Test assumptions	Data checked to verify it meets the assumptions of chosen statistical test	
Normality assumptions (if relevant)	The data was graphed to evaluate the shape of the distribution (graph output)	
	Identified type/level of skewness (numerical output)	
	Identified type/level of kurtosis (numerical output)	
	Based on results can articulate whether data is normally distributed or not	
Generalizability	Sample is checked to ensure it is representative of studied population	
	Sample selection is unbiased	
	Sample size is consistent with the required sample size	
Step 5: Conduct the appropriate analysis		
Conduct analysis	Appropriate test is run	
Significance	Conclusion made about statistical significance	
	If findings were statistically significant, conclusion made about clinical significance	

Training Template

The goal of training should not be to teach basic statistical concepts in isolation; rather the goal for trainers should be to guide health professionals and administrators in the development of critical thinking about statistical concepts. Being able to think critically about statistics will enable practitioners to design simple studies, interpret research, and most importantly to communicate with statistical consultants. To this end, trainers should guide health care professionals and administrators through the process of formulating a research question and hypothesis, designing the study, conducting the analysis, and making conclusions. Rather than teaching the key issues to be aware of in isolation, the understanding of the key issues needs to be made in the context of the framework. Healthcare professionals and administrators should be guided to think of these issues and how they may affect not only the relevant part of the framework, but also the overall statistical process and conclusions. The common data uses that have been previously identified are the most likely scenarios where clinicians and administrators will need to employ statistical thinking, though they are not exhaustive of all the situations that they may encounter. However, once health care professionals and administrators have been taught this process of thinking, it can be applied to any statistical issues that they may encounter.

This approach to teaching applied statistics requires that trainees have basic level knowledge of statistical concepts, such as independent vs. dependent variables, descriptive statistics, and p-values. For trainees who need some refreshers on these concepts, www.statisticshowto.com and the Statistics Learning Centre YouTube channel are great online resources with short videos on key statistical concepts. The textbooks *Statistics for People Who (Think They) Hate Statistics* by Neil J. Salkind and *Fundamental Statistics for the Social and Behavioral Sciences* by Howard T. Tokunaga both explain statistical notions in an approachable manner. *Statistics for People Who (Think They) Hate Statistics* is a particularly easy book to read and serves as a great refresher for those who have not taken or used statistics in some time. Trainers may request that trainees read this book prior to beginning the course. *Statistics for People Who (Think They) Hate Statistics* comes in both SPSS and Excel versions, so if one of these software programs will be used during the training course, trainers should be careful to recommend the corresponding version of the book.

There are a variety of statistical analytical programs that can be used for data analysis. Trainers should select a program that their trainees are familiar with and will have access to after completing the course. If your organization does not emphasize using a specific software program, Microsoft Excel is a good choice. The preprogramed functions as well as the data analysis toolpak have robust functionality, which can be supplemented with online calculators where needed, and Microsoft Excel is readily available in almost every organization.

When training commences, a formal or informal meeting schedule should be established. This may be weekly, bi-weekly, or any interval that works for the trainees. However, stretching the interval out too long could make it more difficult to capitalize on the momentum developed during the sessions. The training process should be to select one of the use cases, present a mock dataset, and walk the trainees through the framework step by step. During the meetings, the trainer should take more of a facilitator approach, guiding the participants to identify and understand the key issues for the relevant part of the framework. Some of the material may necessitate that the trainer lecture or explain concepts, but allowing the participants to discuss the material and come to realizations for themselves is ideal. Depending on the complexity of the section, one session may move through one or more parts of the framework. On the other hand, some of the sections of the framework may take multiple sessions to work through. Below is a sample template for what designing a course or series of courses on applied statistical training could look like (see Table 10.8). The purpose of the template is to provide activities that can help with teaching the five steps to conducting a research study.

Table 10.8 Sample training template

Meeting number	Topic(s)	Activities
Step 1: Develop a primary question and hypotheses		
1	• Course introduction • Statistics review (optional)	Introduce use cases and course structure Discussion about participant expectations Statistics background review if needed
2	• How would you use data? • General questions	Discussion on how they may need to use data to inform their practice Introduce the idea of general research questions Discussion on what general questions they may have Training exercise: Individual brainstorming exercise where they need to list: An area/topic they would be interested in exploring Needs of their current health-care center Barriers to achieving the needs of their health-care center How they think their health-care center could improve Generate a research question based on their list
3	• Fishing • What information do you need to know?	Why do you need definitions? Discussion on how what we want to study must be defined so that it can be measured Discussion about fishing and why it is important to develop a question first Discuss the different foci that could be taken (difference between groups, relationships between variables) Brainstorming about the information that you need to answer this question
4	• Definitions • Hypothesis development	Discussion on why you need to have a specific question (hypothesis) in order to evaluate it Small work groups to determine: How they can test their research question The groups they plan to compare The differences they expect to see in the two groups The time period in which they expect to see the difference
Step 2: Design the study		
5	• Other: variables/ confounders • Measurement scale	Brainstorm about the other information that you need to consider Discuss confounders and how they can affect the study Discussion about different types of variables (nominal, ordinal, interval/ratio) and what type of analysis can be done with them

(continued)

Table 10.8 (continued)

Meeting number	Topic(s)	Activities
6	• Setting the significance level • Type I and type II error	Short video on what is the *p*-value Training exercise: Find visual, memorable ways to teach trainees about the difference between type I and type II error, for example: Type I error: A picture of someone screaming "fire," but there is no fire (false positive) Type II error: A picture of no one screaming "fire," when there is a fire (false negative)
7	• Cause and effect • Study design	Trainer shows Freakonomics short video on spurious correlations Discussion about correlation versus causation Training exercise: Trainer provides scenarios and has the class brainstorm how they could establish cause and effect. What information would they need to do this? List out the different types of study designs List the advantages and disadvantages of each type of study design Compare and contrast study designs Indicate and justify which study design makes the most sense for their proposed study
8	• Clustered data • Test selection	Trainer provides some scenarios where data might be clustered In small groups, trainees will brainstorm ideas of where clustered data may occur in their health care facility's EHR Discussion on different study designs Small work groups: Trainer provides examples of hypotheses, study designs, and statistical tests, and as a group, trainees must match up each hypothesis with the proper study design and statistical test
9	• Generalizability	Discussion on sample size and sample size calculations Discussion on the importance of having a representative sample Small work groups: Trainer provides examples of study results where trainees need to determine if the results can or cannot be generalized Trainer provides a scientific article to each group of trainees where they must determine and justify if the sample was: Representative of studied population Randomly chosen Large enough to conduct their analyses Trainees must indicate the implications of their scientific article not following any of the above rules for sample selection and share with the larger group

(continued)

Table 10.8 (continued)

Meeting number	Topic(s)	Activities
Step 3: Data collection		
10	• Collect data: primary data collection	Discussion about steps in data acquisition through primary collection Discussion on issues to be aware of in data collection (setting up a data management system, standardization of data entry, and standardizing measurements collected)
11	• Collect data: secondary data acquisition	Discussion about steps in data acquisition from secondary source or from EHRs Discussion on what will necessary for data management
Step 4: Prepare the data for analysis		
12	• Descriptive statistics	Discussion about the statistics that can be computed for the types of variables present in the dataset Trainees will use sample data to run descriptive statistics Discussion about descriptive statistics (measures of central tendency, measures of variance, and data distribution) and what they tell you
13	• Data cleaning: missing information, outliers	Trainees will use sample data to run frequencies and create histograms of the variables of interest or be provided with the output by trainer Discussion about issues involved with data cleaning (missing data, outliers, etc.) and how to resolve them Trainees must decide how to handle missing data Trainees must decide how to handle outliers
14	• Test assumptions • Verifying statistical assumptions	Discussion on statistical assumptions Training exercise: Trainer provides the same mock dataset to all trainees Trainees follow along as the trainer walks them through how to check for normality by evaluating skewness, and kurtosis Trainer then provides a different mock dataset to all trainees Trainees must complete the checks for normality by evaluating skewness, and kurtosis on their own Trainees will use the skewness and kurtosis results from the sample data set to determine whether the data is normally distributed Trainees will verify that the assumptions of the chosen test are met
15	• Generalizability	Will ensure that their sample meets criteria established and is generalizable

(continued)

Table 10.8 (continued)

Meeting number	Topic(s)	Activities
Step 5: Conduct the appropriate analysis		
16	• Conducting analysis	Class either uses sample data to run a t-test, or trainer presents output from statistical test Discussion about the results and terms involved (t-test statistic, critical value, *p*-value, etc.)
17	• Interpreting results: statistical significance	Trainer presents information on the methods to determine statistical significance (compare critical value to test statistic or compare *p*-value to chosen level of significance) Discussion about whether or not these results are statistically significant
18	• Interpreting results: clinical significance	Discussion about the difference between statistical and clinical significance Discussion about methods used to determine clinical significance Training exercise: Trainer will divide the class into small groups and provide each group with a set of statistically significant results; trainees need to determine if the results have clinical relevance and provide justification as a team for their position. A spokesperson from each group will share their findings with the larger group, so all can learn
19	• Presentations (optional)	Trainees present their data results and conclusions to the group
20	• Course wrap up	Discussion on the overall conclusions that have been made Discussion about how their thinking changed or what surprised them during the course

Summary

As the use of statistics has moved from an academic setting to a health care setting, health care providers are now expected to make data-based clinical decisions and to be able to demonstrate improvements in patient outcomes. In order to do this, they need to understand not just statistical concepts but how to apply those concepts to the challenges that they face. Traditional statistics training has fallen short in this regard. However, by teaching statistical concepts and data analysis in the applied manner put forth in this chapter, trainees will learn not only how to conduct a study, but more importantly how to think about the problems they face in a critical way. Thus, they are developing not only a new set of analytic skills but more importantly a new way of thinking about and approaching the research questions they encounter.

These critical thinking skills will enable practitioners to visualize and approach clinical challenges in a strategic way, a way that is crucial to the success of the modern-day health care organization.

References

Ford, I., & Norrie, J. (2016). Pragmatic trials. *New England Journal of Medicine, 375*(5), 454–463. doi: 10.1056/NEJMra1510059

George, D., & Mallery, P. (2010). *SPSS for windows step by step: A simple guide and reference 18.0 update* (11th ed.). Boston, MA: Pearson.

Westfall, P. H. (2014). Kurtosis as peakedness, 1905–2014. R.I.P. *The American Statistician, 68*(3), 191–195. doi: 10.1080/00031305.2014.917055

Section IV
Supporting System Changes for Integration

Chapter 11
Workforce Development: Identifying Continuing Education Needs and Programs for Integrated Behavioral Health Training

Colleen Clemency Cordes

While the past decade has been marked by a proliferation of integrated behavioral health clinics and services, there remain few programs specifically designed to promote the skill development and transformation for providers in this field (Mullin & Funderburk, 2013). Recognizing a looming workforce crisis, Blount and Miller (2009) acknowledged that traditional graduate programs, such as psychology and social work, have historically not adequately trained behavioral health clinicians to work in primary care. Central to the work of an integrated behavioral health provider is the ability to collaborate effectively with interdisciplinary teams and identify and understand each team member's unique roles and responsibilities. Interprofessional education (IPE) is an example of a training approach wherein health professionals learn alongside each other to provide collaborative care (Pippet, Moloney-Johns, Jalilibahabadi, & Gren, 2015). Interprofessional education is increasingly being viewed as a central approach to the development of integrated primary care teams. Additionally, while there is no cross-disciplinary consensus on a specific list of competencies for integrated providers, it is recognized that providers must possess the ability to collaborate with others, communicate effectively with patients, and utilize evidence-based practices within the scope of their role on the primary care team (Mullin & Funderburk, 2013). Ensuring that integrated behavioral health providers are prepared to deliver efficient and effective services requires identifying and referring team members to available IPE training opportunities. Additional trainings may be offered in-house to meet the needs of the care team. This chapter is specifically designed for training managers who are responsible for the training that is provided within their organization.

C. C. Cordes (✉)
Integrated Behavioral Health Programs, College of Health Solutions,
Arizona State University, Phoenix, AZ, USA
e-mail: Colleen.Clemency@asu.edu

C. R. Macchi, R. Kessler (eds.), *Training to Deliver Integrated Care*,
https://doi.org/10.1007/978-3-319-78850-0_11

Identifying Existing Training Opportunities

When considering how integrated primary care providers might receive the requisite knowledge, skills, and abilities to function as effective teams, it is critical to ascertain the modality of instructional delivery that might be most appropriate for a given clinic. Both in-person and distance learning opportunities are currently available, and the pros and cons of each delivery mechanism should be considered before determining the appropriate training approach. For example, while providers may prefer to receive intensive hands-on, in-person training, this may be time and cost-prohibitive within the context of a fast-paced clinic and competing provider schedules. Similarly, distance learning may provide an opportunity for providers to receive appropriate knowledge of integrated care, but may not provide the skills-based training necessary to translate this knowledge into clinical practice.

Existing face-to-face programming takes on a variety of forms and formats, all of which should be carefully examined for their appropriateness before adoption. For providers looking for intensive clinical training opportunities, psychology pre- and postdoctoral training experiences exist and provide 1–2 years of supervised clinical experience. The American Psychological Association (APA; https://apa.org) has developed a directory of training programs that offer a specialized focus on primary care; however, such programs are typically focused on the training of psychologists rather than the diverse healthcare providers who work in primary care, and the intensity of time required for such training may not be realistic. In comparison, clinics may choose to bring in established consultation firms such as Mountainview Consulting (www.mtnviewconsulting.com) for the provision on on-the-job training in the Primary Care Behavioral Health (PCBH) model of care, evidence-based treatments such as Focused Acceptance and Commitment Therapy (FfACT), and/or system consultation to assist in the evaluation of training needs, procedural and policy development to promote integration, and program evaluation.

Increasingly, distance-learning programs have been developed to offer educational opportunities with greater convenience. Such programs may be offered either for graduate credit or for continuing education (CE) credits. Existing certificate programs such as the University of Massachusetts Medical School's Center for Integrated Primary Care 36-hour certificate program (http://www.umassmed.edu/cipc) offer attendees synchronous and interactive education and training over the course of 6-day-long trainings. Similar programs exist at a variety of universities, including the University of Michigan's School of Social Work.

The Doctor of Behavioral Health (DBH) program at Arizona State University (https://chs.asu.edu/dbh) is unique in that it provides graduate training in both clinical and management domains of integrated primary care, utilizing both asynchronous and synchronous modalities. Additionally, current DBH students represent a wide range of professionals interested in integrated care, including, but not limited to, social workers, counselors, occupational therapists, healthcare administrators, and individuals working for insurance organizations. In comparison to CE-based training programs, the DBH program requires an internship experience in a primary care or other integrated care environment, and students receive consultation from providers and managers with experience in the healthcare field. While the DBH program is of interest to many master's level providers looking to expand their skills and receive a doctoral degree, the time and cost of such an intensive degree program may not be feasible for many.

Developing In-House Training Opportunities

In some cases, a training manager might be interested in developing original training materials suited to the specific needs of their clinic. Such individuals are encouraged to not start from scratch, but rather look into existing self-study resources to guide their development. Comprehensive lists of such resources are beyond the scope of this chapter but have been reviewed elsewherc (Serrano et al., 2018), including commonly cited texts by Robinson and Reiter (2016), Hunter and colleagues (2017), and Corso and colleagues (2016).

Clinics choosing to develop and implement their own in-services are usually interested to provide training targeted specifically to the identified needs of their providers. Offering in-services assumes that there are qualified individuals within the clinic who have the appropriate knowledge and skills necessary to train other providers. Such in-house training opportunities may include, but are not limited to:, cross-disciplinary didactic experiences such as grand rounds, shadowing of more experienced providers, and/or engaging in process improvement teams.

Considerations for Adopting Workforce Development Programming

Trainers should consider several factors before making a decision to promote the adoption of existing workforce development programming or to develop their own in-services. Thoughtful consideration of the following questions is recommended to ensure efficient and effective training for all those involved:

1) Who is the audience we are trying to train? Are they already on-the-job, or are we training them before launching into services?

It is essential to determine not only *who* you are looking to train (i.e., physicians, behavioral health providers, medical assistants, front desk staff, or all of the above), but also *what* your expectations are for each team member once they have acquired the skills. While IPE experiences foster broad approaches to collaboration, specialized training based on an individual's background may be needed for some of the team members. For example, a behavioral health provider may benefit from basic training around the medical pathophysiology of diabetes, whereas this information would be unnecessary for medical providers. It is critical to ensure that training opportunities are tailored to the needs of the specific audience. Similarly, as noted above, understanding *when* training will be provided during the professional lifecycle might also dictate the type of educational opportunities that are pursued. Questions about timing include:

- Are you providing basic training to providers new to the field or clinical environment?
- Are you providing retraining of existing skills sets?
- Are you intending to deepen and expand the competencies of the team?

Answers to each of these questions necessitate a different approach to training and should be considered thoughtfully when establishing "fit" between provider/clinic needs and training program.

2) What do I want providers to know/be able to accomplish upon completion of this training?

Depending upon the training goals, addressing a given population influences the kind of programming to pursue. For example, for clinics/providers hoping to gain basic knowledge, asynchronous, didactic online programming may sufficiently meet their needs, as knowledge can readily be assessed by basic learning assessments such as quizzes. In comparison, higher level learning objectives that require skill acquisition and practice such as skills in motivational interviewing may necessitate interactive opportunities for practice, whether through role play or standardized patients (see Bloom's taxonomy for more information about cognitive learning objectives, http://www.learningandteaching.info/learning/bloomtax.htm).

3) What resources do I have (financial, staffing, time)?

In an age where clinics are increasingly under-resourced for their needs, it is critical to determine the nature and amount of resources available for pursuing workforce development opportunities. For example, while intensive graduate education may be the desired route to ensure high-level skill acquisition, the costs associated with pursing this kind of program might be prohibitive. Similarly, education aimed at skill acquisition often requires greater time and staffing than knowledge-based training, as providers will need ongoing feedback about their burgeoning competencies, and regular practice of these skills. For many of these reasons, distance learning certificates, which tend to be lower in cost and require less time and clinic staffing, may be desirable; in such cases, focus on skill development may need to be sacrificed due to limited resources.

4) What model of integration is our clinic looking to adopt/has adopted already?

Many established programs have as their framework for training a preference for a particular model of integrated care. It is necessary that a clinic/provider pursuing such training opportunities determines if the model put forth in the particular training aligns with their clinic's needs. While many existing programs have focused, for example, on the PCBH model of care delivery, this may not be appropriate for a traditional behavioral health clinic looking to integrate primary care into their offering ("reverse or bidirectional integration"). For these clinics, consultation or in-services delivered by experts with knowledge of this particular model of care may provide more robust and appropriate training opportunities than attempting to adopt an inappropriate model of care.

5) Are continuing medical education (CMEs) necessary?

While it may be preferable to be able to provide continuing education to those participating in an educational opportunity, this is not always feasible or realistic, particularly in the case of interprofessional in-services, wherein multiple types of CEs (e.g., physician, nursing, psychologist, social work) may be required and a clinic may not already be an authorized provider of CEs. While becoming a provider of continuing education credits is certainly a possibility (http://www.accme.org/cme-providers/first-time-applicant), it is not always realistic. As such, in cases where the provision of CMEs is necessary for provider engagement, partnering with established CME providers and/or exploring programming that already offers CMEs may be preferred.

References

Blount, F. A., & Miller, B. F. (2009). Addressing the workforce crisis in integrated primary care. *Journal of Clinical Psychology in Medical Settings, 16*, 113–119.

Corso, K. A., Hunter, C. L., Dahl, O., Kallenberg, G. A., & Manson, L. (2016). *Integrating behavioral health into the medical home: A rapid implementation guide*. Phoenix, MD: Greenbranch publishing.

Hunter, C., Goodie, J., Oordt, M., & Dobmeyer, A. (2017). *Integrated behavioral health in primary care: Step-by-step guidance for assessment and intervention* (2nd ed.): American Psychological Association.

Mullin, D. J., & Funderburk, J. S. (2013). Implementing clinical interventions in integrated behavioral health settings: Best practices and essential elements. In M. R. Talen & A. Burke Valeras

(Eds.), *Integrated behavioral health in primary care: Evaluating the evidence, identifying the essentials* (pp. 273–297). New York: Springer.

Pippet, K., Moloney-Johns, A., Jalilibahabadi, S., & Gren, L. H. (2015). Collaboration versus competition: An interprofessional education experience. *Family Medicine, 47*(4), 298–301.

Robinson, P. J., & Reiter, J. T. (2016). *Behavioral consultation in primary care: A guide to integrating services (2nd Ed.).* New York, NY: Springer.

Serrano, N., Cordes, C., Cubic, B., & Daub, S. (2018). The state and future of the primary care behavioral health model of service delivery workforce. *Journal of Clinical Psychology in Medical Settings, 25*, 157–168. https://www.ncbi.nlm.nih.gov/pubmed/28508140

Chapter 12
Ethical Integrated Healthcare

Lesley Manson

Chapter overview	
Domains	*Healthcare delivery improvements and efficiencies* *Integrated healthcare workforce training*
Key points	*Comprehensive overview of current legal, ethical, and professional issues essential to integrated care settings. Examination and exploration of multiple healthcare professional guilds and association ethics and legalities and federal regulations. Understanding and application of respect, autonomy, justice, non-maleficence, and beneficence. Improving outcomes and safety through reporting guidelines and integrated ethical practice. Review, ethical decision-making, and utilization of electronic health records and medical technology for integrated care. Utilization of decision-making and problem-solving tool to resolve interprofessional legal, ethical, and professional challenges in integrated healthcare systems*
Student learning objectives (SLOs)	1. *Evaluate the philosophical and theoretical underpinnings of ethical decision-making* 2. *Summarize the essential features of medical and behavioral ethics* 3. *Identify, evaluate, and assemble legal, ethical, and professional principles most essential for the clinical practice of integrated behavioral healthcare* 4. *Evaluate the challenges that may arise as a result of differences in behavioral health and medical ethical codes* 5. *Explore common ethical issues arising in medical care settings and discriminate the best process to address* 6. *Examine and evaluate ethical dilemmas arising from clinical practice with patients from diverse populations* 7. *Review and evaluate the emerging principles of medical ethics applied to electronic medical records, eHealth, mHealth, and other emerging health technologies*

L. Manson (✉)
Integrated Behavioral Health Programs, College of Health Solutions, Arizona State University, Phoenix, AZ, USA
e-mail: lesley.manson@asu.edu

C. R. Macchi, R. Kessler (eds.), *Training to Deliver Integrated Care*,
https://doi.org/10.1007/978-3-319-78850-0_12

Chapter overview	
Instructional strategies	*Lecture, discussion, video/media, assigned readings, role play, coaching, and presentations*
Evaluating learning	*Quizzes, written ethical case review assignments, grading discussions, presentations, and final examination*

Historical Perspectives on Ethical Standards and Practice

Ethical, legal, and professional issues have evolved by different professional guild viewpoints (Botes, 2000a, 2000b; Wynia, Kishore, & Belar, 2014; Rolfsenm, 2010). Philosophical positions followed moral theories and generated aspirational principles guiding ethical decision-making. Guilds created ethical codes, guidelines, and standards of behavior supported by enforceable standards. Further, guilds guided state agencies toward creating legal statutes, defining required professional decision-making. Training programs traditionally provided guild guided ethical and legal instruction. Interprofessional perspective and understanding was generally lacking.

Presently, an interprofessional understanding and approach to ethical training is essential in a rapidly evolving integrated world of healthcare where team-based, interprofessional care is becoming the standard of healthcare. Behavioral/mental, medical, and allied healthcare professionals are being asked to work in collaborative team-based care. Understanding unique laws (i.e., legal statutes and reporting requirements), ethical perspectives and challenges, and guild principles of each team member is crucial. This integrated perspective allows for professionals to build an understanding of each other's ethical roles, responsibilities, moral perspectives, and legal obligations as part of the care delivery team (Botes, 2000a, 2000b; Lau, 2010). In addition, an integrated perspective to teaching and training provides a framework for practical application of team-based, legal, and ethical decision-making.

Principles of Ethical Practice

The first step toward developing a curriculum to address an integrated ethical and legal perspective is knowledge of the differing guilds and their associated codes of conduct, guidelines, and statutes. Learners should be at least aware of and familiar with the ethical guidelines of the American Psychological Association, American Medical Association, American Psychiatric Association, American Nurses Association, National Association of Social Workers, American Association for Marriage and Family Therapy, American College of Healthcare Executives, and

Table 12.1 Principles of ethical practice

Principle	Theory alignment	Definition
Respect for persons/autonomy	Duty-based ethical theory	Acknowledge a person's right to make choices, to hold views, and to take actions based on personal values and beliefs
Justice	Duty-based ethical theory	Treat others equitably, distribute benefits/burdens fairly
Non-maleficence (do no harm)	Outcome-based ethical theory	Obligation not to inflict harm intentionally; "first, do no harm"
Beneficence (do good)	Outcome-based ethical theory	Provide benefits to persons and contribute to their welfare. Refers to an action done for the benefit of others

Interprofessional Education Collaborative (IPEC). Instructors are encouraged to choose three to four guild guidelines including those from IPEC, for in-depth review, education, and training on how to integrate the different perspectives. The mission of IPEC is to "promote, encourage, and support efforts to prepare future health professionals so that they enter the workforce ready for interprofessional collaborative practice that helps to ensure the health of individuals and populations" (IPEC, 2016). Over 14 medical associations/guilds are aligned with IPEC and collaborate on developing the IPEC core competencies in interprofessional education. In addition, the World Health Organization (WHO) has supported a framework for interprofessional education and collaborative practice in healthcare (WHO, 2010).

As we train learners to be familiar with the legal and ethical interdisciplinary codes of conduct, guidelines, and statutes, they will develop a knowledge and sense of shared and conflictual roles and responsibilities. This will assist them in building a cross-discipline approach to understanding and addressing ethical decision-making. For the instructor, using an interdisciplinary approach helps to broaden the scope and increase momentum of the transformation of interprofessional integrated education.

Learners should be encouraged to explore the philosophical underpinnings of moral decision-making through a multidimensional, integrated perspective. The philosophers, Tom Beauchamp and Jim Childress, proposed four principles that provide a set of moral pillars for applying values and judgments to applied practice: respect for persons/autonomy, justice, non-maleficence, and beneficence (Cook, Mavroudis, Jacobs, Mavroudis, & Miracle, 2016; Lustig, 2013; Miracle, 2016). Continual consideration of these principles supports practitioners' efforts to balance and align duties with patient-centered outcomes (Miracle, 2016). Further, through a cross-discipline approach to ethical decision-making, health professionals are reinforced to develop and maintain a climate of mutual respect and shared values, linking principles to practice (Table 12.1).

Principles of Interprofessional Ethical Practice

There are many shared principles for integrated care professionals. As learners become familiar with the key principles of ethical practice (i.e., respect for persons/autonomy, justice, non-maleficence, and beneficence), they can begin to identify the guild-specific codes of conduct and ethical standards that link to these principles. For example, the American Psychological Association and American Medical Association both align their ethical codes of conduct with these four principles of ethical practice. Identifying diverging values is critical in an integrated interprofessional decision-making approach. Teaching exercises should follow an integrated, interprofessional approach (see Table 12.2) that applies each principle to ethical decision-making. The integrated decision-making tool can be applied to integrated care professional case reviews. Learners can utilize the tool to explore guild-specific and shared moral principles for team-based decision-making. Three categories of questions address the four principles, guild-specific inquiry, and exploration of legal and professional perspectives in integrated care. Addressing each question elucidates diverging and conflicting legal, ethical, and professional codes, values, and principles through challenging the learner to identify their own and other team member's views. Using tools for ethical decision-making, which require interdisciplinary critical thinking, enhances transparency and collaboration in teams through the identification of parity, mutual goals and understanding, and shared accountability. Trainers may use this tool (see Table 12.2) in three primary ways: (1) in a role play that assists the learner in walking through an integrated ethical, legal, and/or professional challenge while ensuring they complete each column, what the learner considers and what they believe and can identify through research, their interprofessional team member must consider and assist with identifying a final integrated decision, combining the practice ethics, interests, legal aspects, and professional considerations of all parties involved; (2) as a supervision tool guiding the learner through this process; and/or (3) as a consultation ethical decision-making tool, integrated team members can utilize together to ensure they ask each other important questions (motives, behaviors, legalities, confidentiality, scope of practice, practice ethics, professional, and consequences and outcomes) and learn from each other to end with an integrated decision. Table 12.3 walks through an integrated team members' consultation together as they explore an ethical and legal challenge. It is essential that trainers challenge learners to walk through each column regardless of their perspective of the application or their views on which elements pertain to their legal, ethical, or professional situation.

Ethical Challenges of Team-Based Integrated Practice

Identifying appropriate integrated legal, ethical, and professional cases for review is challenging. Case examples can be generated through reviewing the principle-integrated care challenges identified in the literature and surrounding the Quadruple Aim of healthcare (see Table 12.4) (Bodenheimer & Sinsky, 2014; Runyan,

Table 12.2 Integrated ethical, legal, and professional decision-making chart

	What I know *Witnessed, ethics, situation, legal, professional (consider guild)*	**Others involved (team)** *Witnessed, ethics, situation, legal, professional (consider multi-guild and professional perspectives)*	**Integrated care decision-making** *Specific choices and required actions; next steps; application for individual, team, and patient; shared decision-making*
Motives *Why ask question?* *What is happening?* *Were motivations good?* *Was there harm?* *Benefits and burdens?*			
Behaviors (refrain from interpretation) *What happened?* *What is happening?* *Was there respect for autonomy? Challenge the definition of autonomy to include personal, cultural, community, and familial viewpoints.* *Was the person/situation treated equitably?*			
Legalities *Legal considerations; statutes*			
Confidentiality *Who, what, when, where, and why; need*			
Scope of practice *Limitations* *Strengths* *Roles and responsibilities*			
Practice ethics *Specific standards or recommendations*			
Professional: *Cultural, power, business, financial concerns?*			
Consequences and outcomes *What has happened as a result?* *What would I like to happen? What will happen?* *Was there harm? Good?* *What can I control/do?*			
Additional info			

Table 12.3 Integrated ethical, legal, and professional decision-making tool

	What I know *Witnessed, ethics, situation, legal, professional (consider guild)*	**Others involved (team)** *Witnessed, ethics, situation, legal, professional (consider multi-guild and professional perspectives)*	**Integrated care decision-making** *Specific choices and required actions; next steps; application for individual, team, and patient; shared decision-making*
Motives *Why ask question?* *What is happening?* *Were motivations good?* *Was there harm?* *Benefits and burdens?*	Query on whether need to report domestic violence (DV)	Query on who is required to report domestic violence to police	
Behaviors (refrain from interpretation) *What happened?* *What is happening?* *Was there respect for autonomy?* *Challenge the definition of autonomy to include personal, cultural, community, and familial viewpoints* *Was the person/situation treated equitably?*	Patient presented to clinic with bruising and lacerations on the face and body. Pt received treatment from primary care provider related to injuries. Pt disclosed in warm handoff to BH support that injuries were result of domestic violence	Pt requested that injuries are not reported to police	To respect autonomy and the personal viewpoints of the pt., we must share with the pt. the legal obligations and plan to report
Legalities *Legal considerations; statutes*	BH has no legal obligation to report domestic violence due to pt. and does not meet criteria for adult protective services nor has children in home	PCP reviews suspicious injury protocol and reporting guidelines for their state	PCP is legally obligated in their state to report the DV due to treating the injuries
Confidentiality *Who, what, when, where, and why; need*	Obtain verbal consent to share information with pcp. Further, pt. is in a team-based integrated healthcare site with shared charting and confidentiality	Obtain verbal consent to share information with pcp. Further, pt. is in a team-based integrated healthcare site with shared charting and confidentiality	

Scope of practice *Limitations* *Strengths* *Roles and responsibilities*	N/A	N/A	
Practice ethics *Specific standards or recommendations*	Reviewed BH ethical codes. Identified need to communicate with pt. if need to report DV to police	Identified need to communicate with pt. if need to report DV to police	Plan to discuss the reporting guidelines with the pt. and offer to call with pt. present
Professional *Cultural, power, business, financial concerns?*	N/A	N/A	
Consequences and outcomes *What has happened as a result?* *What would I like to happen? What will happen?* *Was there harm? Good?* *What can I control/do?*	Pt is in exam room waiting for primary care provider to return with further guidance Concerns of pt. safety	Concerned pt. will not return to practice and pcp for care	Plan to prepare a safety plan, crisis information, review police reporting, and discuss as a team approach with the pt. in exam room. Plan for pcp to take lead due to relationship
Additional info		Long-standing pt. of pcp	

Table 12.4 Legal, ethical, and professional case topics

Integrated care topic	Application	Healthcare aim
Billing and coding	Ensuring appropriate ethical and legal billing, coding, and documentation; reviewing state and federal regulations	Reducing the per capita cost of healthcare
Confidentiality and Health Insurance Portability and Accountability Act (HIPAA) regulations	Review of HIPAA regulations and challenging preconceptions of confidentiality in team-based care; reviewing state and federal regulations	*Improving the patient experience of care*
Consent	Ensuring consent for team-based care	Improving the patient experience of care
Evidence-based treatments and interventions	Assurance and review of interventions and treatment which aligns with evidence for all professionals and is not conflicting in prescription	Improving the health of populations Reducing the per capita cost of healthcare Improving the patient experience of care Improving the healthcare team's experience
Medical errors	Identification of medical errors, addressing with patients and families, and exploration of communication errors as primary cause. Review of shared communication techniques	Improving the health of populations Reducing the per capita cost of healthcare Improving the patient experience of care Improving the healthcare team's experience
Medical necessity	Review of integrated healthcare interventions following medical necessity	Improving the health of populations
Roles and responsibilities	Identification of each team member's distinct role, responsibilities, and areas of flexibility within the care team	Improving the health of populations Reducing the per capita cost of healthcare Improving the patient experience of care Improving the healthcare team's experience
Reporting requirements (e.g., child and adult regulations, infectious disease)	Exploration of mandated reporting statutes based on professional guild and license (e.g., reporting domestic violence wound care by medical providers and confidentiality implications for behavioral providers, new infectious disease)	Improving the health of populations Improving the patient experience of care Improving the healthcare team's experience
Scope of practice	Areas of limitation related to professional license and training. Exploration of the reach of license and training in integrated-/team-based care	Improving the health of populations Reducing the per capita cost of healthcare Improving the patient experience of care Improving the healthcare team's experience
Technology in healthcare	Ensuring consent, application, review, and recommendation of appropriate use of electronic medical records and mHealth	Improving the health of populations Reducing the per capita cost of healthcare Improving the patient experience of care Improving the healthcare team's experience

Robinson, & Gould, 2013; Saarni, Parmanne, & Halila, 2008). These challenges may be divided into the main areas of consent, confidentiality and Health Insurance Portability and Accountability Act (HIPAA) regulations, billing and coding, medical necessity, medical errors, technology in healthcare, reporting requirements, scope of practice, roles and responsibilities, and evidence-based treatments and interventions (Elger, 2009; Hudgins, Rose, Arnault, & Fifield, 2013; Institute of Medicine, 2001; Kanzler, Goodie, Hunter, Glotfelter, & Bodart, 2013; Lillemoen & Pedersen, 2012; Reiter & Runyan, 2013; Runyan et al., 2013). A review of these main areas aligned with the healthcare aim and area of challenge is provided in Table 12.4.

Designing Training to Address Interprofessional, Team-Based, Integrated Practice

Training focused on ethics can improve behaviors, moral decision-making, and reasoning (Lau, 2010). A primary recommendation is to create activities that emphasize application and generalization through the use of healthcare scenarios. Once the topics are identified, activities may entail knowledge assessments (quizzes and tests), integrated case explorations (assigning each student to a different professional perspective and guild on an integrated team), formal discussions, and individuals and/or team-based presentations. A challenge may be to invite learners to build a cross-disciplinary or interprofessional code of ethics for integrated practices. For a review of suggested applied assignments, see Table 12.5. Enck (2014) also provides an applied six-step framework for legal, ethical, and professional applied learning. The six-step framework may be utilized in applied assignments and evaluations for learners. Enck's (2014) steps include information (obtaining information relevant to the patient's medical and behavioral history inclusive of cross-disciplinary goals of care, treatment planning, and consultations), identification (identification and assessment of ethical, legal, professional, and social issues and alignment of the interprofessional team member, service, or department for addressing), clarification (communication with the integrated team members, patient, and their support to ensure understanding; defining of ethical, legal, or professional concerns; and next steps), assessment (assessing cross-disciplinary considerations and patient's preferences, interests, values, and quality of life), recommendation (final multidisciplinary recommendation to the team and patient/supports delivered in a way all parties can understand), and documentation (shared medical record documentation of the team's decisions; ethical, legal, or professional challenges and management; follow-up; decision-making; and recommendations). Learner assignments and evaluations may be designed to ensure these areas of application are completed.

Table 12.5 Suggested applied assignments

Assignment type	Team-based integrated challenge
Discussions	Pose various questions related to ethical, legal, and professional quandary and exploration Provide various professional articles which conflict with recommendations to illustrate interdisciplinary team challenges Require learners to respond to the questions and readings through online discussions, formal debates, or in-class presentations targeted at cross-disciplinary/interprofessional shared decision-making and problem-solving
Groups	Assign learners into groups reviewing specific professional ethical codes Require learners to identify shared roles and responsibilities and develop a cross-disciplinary or interprofessional code of ethics for integrated practices
Integrated cases	Assign learners to a specific healthcare license type and association Provide a scenario related to treatment planning and continuity of care Learners will be required to identify their scope of practice, roles and responsibilities, and evidence-based treatments/interventions which elucidate team-based care planning, shared goals, and provision of care
Knowledge assessments (quizzes and tests)	Create multiple choice- and scenario-based questions challenging learners to work through consent, reporting, and HIPAA regulations
Presentations	Encourage learners to identify specific integrated care challenges (e.g., technology, medical errors, medical necessity, billing, and coding), a specific integrated care team (e.g., behavioral health provider, medical provider, allied health, and nursing), and review each professional code and legal requirement related to the challenge Ensure the learners utilize the integrated ethical, legal, and professional decision-making chart and illustrate the ethical principle (autonomy, justice, non-maleficence, and maleficence)
Videos/media/ role plays	Using video and patient simulations allows for learners to explore and apply ethical principles, review cases through multiple professional lenses, and explore theoretical underpinnings of ethical decision-making

Cultural Dimensions of Integrated Team-Based Training

A comprehensive ethical training program addresses the range of cultural issues related to integrated team-based practice. Instruction needs to include attention to issues focused on special populations and applied integrated care topics such as geriatrics, pediatrics, military, tribal, transgender, religion, culture, identity, disability, technology-based, coding/billing/documentation, confidentiality, medical procedure decision-making, shared decision-making, and stigma. Challenging learners' views applied to specific cases is essential. Instructors are encouraged to consider identifying specific integrated healthcare case examples focused on special populations for review. Consider challenging cases such as end of life decision-making, concerns and/or refusal of team-based behavioral healthcare due to stigma, limited medical and general literacy, cultural and religious concerns with medical procedures, limited English proficiency and use of interpreters, and readiness for hormone replacement therapy in gender identity. Learners need to (1) evaluate interprofessional ethical codes (compare and contrast), (2) apply statutes and (3) the four principles, and (4) identify specific distinct interprofessional challenges and dilemmas. Consider using the *integrated ethical, legal, and professional decision-making chart* (see Table 12.2). Challenge teams of students to work together and align themselves with various guilds and professional identities and explore common ethical viewpoints to discriminate best practice for shared decision-making.

Evaluating Learning

A fundamental instructional task is to evaluate the impact and proficiency of integrated ethical decision-making and applied performance. Instructors are encouraged to build rubrics addressing the learners' ability to introduce an ethical, legal, and professional dilemma (who, what, and why), how a dilemma is typically addressed without shared integrated team-based decision-making (addressing consequences of individualized decision making in integrated care), and how the dilemma is resolved through shared multidisciplinary decision-making and review. It is important for the learners to examine and demonstrate proficiency in HIPAA regulations and cross-disciplinary state reporting guidelines and statutes. As a reminder, learners must be consistently reminded to apply a multidisciplinary framework and challenge them to explore beyond their own default lens, ethics, and professional expectations. Practical application of this learning, as opposed to abstract philosophical theorizing, is critical to ensure an integrated care workforce is ready for the demands of an integrated healthcare system focused on team-based problem-solving, decision-making, and provision of care.

Conclusion

As integrated team-based healthcare becomes the predominate form of healthcare delivery to meet the demands of the Quadruple Aim, we must prepare the healthcare workforce to be competent, ethically sound, and prepared to work effectively within interprofessional teams (Institute of Medicine, 2001). Strong training in legal, ethical, and professional decision-making from a multidisciplinary lens is essential. Through following these practical recommendations and guidelines and using the applied decision-making tools and assignments focused on integrated case topics, our healthcare workforce will demonstrate readiness for team-based practice transformation.

References

Botes, A. (2000a). A comparison between the ethics of justice and the ethics of care. *Journal of Advanced Nursing, 32*(5), 1071–1075.
Botes, A. (2000b). An integrated approach to ethical decision-making in the health team. *Journal of Advanced Nursing, 32*(5), 1076–1082.
Bodenheimer, T & Sinsky, C. (2014). From triple to quadruple aim: Care of patient requires care of the provider. *Annals of Family Medicine, 12*(6), 574–576. https://doi.org/10.1370/afm.1713.
Cook, T., Mavroudis, C. D., Jacobs, J. P., Mavroudis, C., & Miracle, V. A. (2016). The Belmont report. The triple crown of research ethics. *Dimensions of Critical Care Nursing, 35*(4), 223–228. https://doi.org/10.1097/DCC.0000000000000186.
Elger, B. S. (2009). Violations of medical confidentiality: Opinions of primary care physicians. *British Journal of General Practice.* 10.339/bjgp09X472647. 59(567): e344–e352. https://doi.org/10.3399/bjgp09X472647
Enck, G. (2014). Six step framework for ethical decision making. *Journal of Health Services Research & Policy, 19*(1), 62–64.
Hudgins, C., Rose, S., Arnault, S., & Fifield, P. (2013). Navigating the legal and ethical foundations of informed consent, and confidentiality in IPC. *Families, Systems & Health, 31*(1), 9–19.
Institute of Medicine. (2001). *Crossing the quality chasm: A new health system for the twenty-first century.* Washington, DC: National Academies Press.
Interprofessional Education Collaborative. (2016). *Core competencies for interprofessional collaborative practice: 2016 update.* Washington, DC: Interprofessional Education Collaborative.
Kanzler, K., Goodie, J. L., Hunter, C. L., Glotfelter, M. A., & Bodart, J. J. (2013). From colleague to patient: Ethical challenges in IPC. *Families, Systems & Health, 31*(1), 41–48.
Lau, C. L. L. (2010). A step forward: Ethics education matters! *Journal of Business Ethics, 92*(4), 565–584. https://doi.org/10.1007/s10551-009-0173-2.
Lillemoen, L., & Pedersen, R. (2012). Ethical challenges and how to develop ethics support in primary care. *Nursing Ethics*, 1–13. https://doi.org/10.1177/0969733012452687.
Lustig, A. B. (2013). Dignity in the discourses of bioethics. *An interdisciplinary journal, 96*(3), 297–314.
Miracle, V.A. (2016, July/August). *The belmont report. The triple crown of research ethics.* Educational Dimension. https://doi.org/10.1097/DCC.0000000000000186.
Reiter, J., & Runyan, C. (2013). The ethics of complex relationships in primary care behavioral health. *Families, Systems, & Health, 31*, 20–27.
Rolfsenm, M. L. (2010). Ethics in the primary care office. *Journal of Louisiana State Medical Society, 162*, 26–32.
Runyan, C., Robinson, P., & Gould, D. A. (2013). Ethical issues facing providers in collaborative primary care settings. *Families, Systems, & Health, 31*(1), 1–8.
Saarni, S., Parmanne, P., & Halila, R. (2008). Ethically problematic treatment decisions: A physician survey. *Bioethics, 22*(2), 121–129.
World Health Organization (2010). Framework for action on interprofessional education and collaborative practice. Retreived from: http://www.who.int/hrh/nursing_midwifery/en/.
Wynia, M. K., Kishore, S. P., & Belar, C. D. (2014). A unified code of ethics for health professional. Insights from an IOM workshop. *JAMA, 311*(8), 799–800. https://doi.org/10.1001/jama.2014.504.

Index

A

Accountable Care Organization (ACO), 139
Advancing Integrated Mental Health Solutions (AIMS), 19
Agency for Healthcare Research and Quality (AHRQ), 17
Alternative payment models (APM), 121
American Medical Association, 216
American Psychological Association (APA), 25, 162, 166, 208, 216
Applied assignments, 221, 222
A3 Report, 86, 91, 94

B

Behavioral consultation, 19
Behavioral health (BH)
  carve-in and carve-outs approaches, 5
  clinicians, 5
Behavioral health consultant (BHC), 21, 121
Behavioral health ethics, 222
Behavioral Health Practitioners (BHP), 42
Behavioral health provider, 113
Behavioral health workforce, 117
Behavioral healthcare paradigm (BHP), 27
Behavioral medicine, 115, 117
BHP skill development
  performance evaluation tool, 168–170
  performance metrics, 171
  template development, 173, 174
Big data, 4
Billing codes and reimbursement, 139, 140
Biomedical data
  blood pressure, 191
  cluster, 184
  diabetes, 190
  medical settings, 178
Biopsychosocial approach, 164
Biopsychosocial model, 52
Biopsychosocial model of care (BPS), 16
Biostatistics, *see* Biomedical data
Business case
  BHP, 121
  CoCM, 121, 122
  comparison of competencies, 125
  cost, 126
  financial sustainability, 120
  in-person training, 133
  integrated behavioral health, 120
  measurement and evaluation, 132
  online learning, 132
  PCBH, 121
  pro forma, 122
  ROI, 126
  training and skill acquisition
    calculating program costs, 126, 127
    category, 126
    pro forma, 129, 131
    revenue, 128, 131
    ROI, 130, 131
Business plan
  appendix, 154
  company description, 149
  competition, 150, 151
  core competencies, 147, 148
  executive summary, 148
  financial projections, 154
  grading rubric, 145, 146
  industry analysis and trends, 149
  management and organization, 153
  marketing plan, 151

C. R. Macchi, R. Kessler (eds.), *Training to Deliver Integrated Care*,
https://doi.org/10.1007/978-3-319-78850-0

Business plan (*cont.*)
operations, 152
risk assessment, 151
risks, 154
sales strategy, 152
social responsibility and sustainability, 153
strategic position, 151
target market, 150
technology, 153

C
Care Continuum Alliance (CCA), 69
Care delivery, vii, 38
Care manager, 19
Centers for Medicare and Medicaid Services (CMS), 19
Chronic care management, 67, 70
Chronic Care Model, 18
Collaborative Care Model (CoCM), 91, 121, 122, 124, 126, 133
BHP, 27
care manager, 19
CMS, 19
description, 18
DIAMOND study, 22
IMPACT, 18
Katon group, 19
PCBH model, 22
RCT, 19
Collaborative Family Healthcare Association (CFHA), 22
Colocated therapy model, 17
Common procedural terminology (CPT), 70
Communication (CC), 108
Comprehensive training programs, 8
Confounder, 182, 183
Continuing education (CE), 208, 209
Continuing medical education (CMEs), 211
Continuous quality improvement (CQI), 6
Control charts, 85, 86, 93
Core competencies
behavioral health, 42
clinical, 43, 45
financial, 42, 44, 45
operational, 43, 45
PHM, 71
skills, 41
staff competencies, 42
Cost-effective, 68, 69, 71, 74
Costs
BHP, 131
competencies, 127
financial sustainability, 120
post-intervention utilization, 136
predictive modeling, 122
pre-intervention utilization, 136
program/intervention, 136
revenue, 120
Cost savings, 139
Council for Six Sigma Certification, 87
Cultural issues, 222

D
Data acquisition
codebook, 189
EHR, 188, 189
Data analysis
clustered data, 184–185
histogram, 189
missing information, 190
outlier, 190
skewness, 190
statistical analytical programs, 198, 202
statistical assumptions, 191
toolpak, 198
Degree Program Discussion Board Rubric, 134–136
Degree training programs
APA, 162, 166
barriers, 165
BH, 163
BHP, 163, 164
evaluation tool, 167
performance metrics, 171
financial option, 164
internet-based training, 163
IPE, 166
performance metrics, 167
postdoctoral fellowship for psychologists, 162
primary care settings, 163
self-management activities, 164
skill acquisition, 166, 167
Depression treatment, 117
Determinants of health, 67, 68, 77
DIAMOND study, 22
Doctor of Behavioral Health (DBH), 24, 208
Doctors of osteopathic medicine (DOs), 16

E
Educational programming
CEs, 211
distance-learning, 208
interprofessional in-services, 211

Electronic health records (EHRs), 4, 69, 96, 178, 179
Electronic medical record (EMR), vii
Engagement, 77
Entrepreneurship
business plan, 148
course, 154, 157–159
and education, 144
measurement, 155
nursing, 144
performance barriers, 147
SWOT analysis, 156
VC panels, 147
Ethics
integrated care professionals, 216, 218–219
IPEC, 215
principles, 215
standards and practice, 214
team-based integrated practice, 216, 220
Evaluation template, 196–197
Evidence-based practice, 163, 164

F
Fast-paced clinic, 208
Fee-for-service (FFS) model, 80, 120
Financial implications, 61
Financial management
cost savings, 120
generating sufficient revenue, 120
microsimulation model, 122
PCBH and CoCM, 122
Fishing, 181
Five As model, 48
5 Rs framework
care delivery research, 7
definition, 7
Focused Acceptance and Commitment Therapy (FACT), 208

G
Generalizability, 186, 191
Grading Rubric, 137–139

H
Hawaii Project, 16
Health Insurance Portability and Accountability Act (HIPAA), 221
Health maintenance organization (HMO), 180
Health saving accounts (HSA), 180
Health-care data
clinical decisions, 202
hypothesis, 178
statistical issues, 178, 179, 181, 197, 198
Healthcare delivery, 6
Healthcare management business, 6
Hispanic individuals, 186, 188
Hypothesis testing, 180, 181

I
Improving Mood–Promoting Access to Collaborative Treatment (IMPACT), 18, 19
In-house training, 207, 209
Institute for Healthcare Improvement (IHI), 87
Institute of Medicine (IOM), 19, 20
Integrated behavioral health (IBH) model
American Psychological Association, 24
BHP, 27
clinics and services, 207
CoCM, 25
DBH, 24
design stage, 26
developing stages, 26
Donabedian's dimensions, quality of care, 25
historical shifts, 15
IBH training, 23–25
IPE, 207
management competencies, 124
meta-theoretical approach, 23
SAMHSA-HRSA, 25
strategies, 28–29
training manuals, 23
Integrated care, 104, 107, 112
cultural issues, 222
Integrated ethics, 215, 216, 218–219
Integrated Health Care (IHC), 42
Integrated primary care
DBH, 208
Integrated team-based training
assessment rubrics, 52
behavioral health, 42
care delivery, 38
clinical, 43
core competencies, 41
evaluation phase, 46–49
financial, 42, 44
implementation phase, 46–48
interconnected training phases, 49
linked program and course, 53
objectives, involvement and outcome, 40
operational, 43

Integrated team-based training (*cont.*)
participation, 39–41
preparation phase, 46, 47
principles, 46
responsibilities, 39, 40
roles, 38–39
skill set, 37
staff competencies, 42
whole-person care, 52
workforce plan, 50–51
Integration levels, 6–7
Integration model selection
PIP domain, 27
structure-process-outcomes, 25
International Association for Six Sigma Certification (IASSC), 87
Interprofessional decision-making, 217–219, 223
Interprofessional education (IPE), 105, 163, 166, 207
Interprofessional education and competency (IPEC), 38, 112, 115, 117, 215
Interprofessional ethics, 216, 218–219
Interprofessional teams, 68, 70, 72
Interprofessional training, 41, 43, 46, 55
Intrapreneurship, 144

K
Key performance indicators (KPIs), 87
Kurtosis
design phase, 193
equivalent nonparametric tests, 194
parametric tests, 194

L
Lean Six Sigma
A3 Report, 86, 94
barriers, 87
BCH, 88
causes of waste, 85
components, 81
control charts, 85, 86, 93
data visualization tools, 81
define value, 82
DOWNTIME, 82
error-proofing, 84
establish flow, 83
IASSC, 87
IHI, 85, 87
implement pull, 84
managers and stakeholders, 88
measurement and evaluation, 92, 95
PCMH, 81
PDSA, 85, 91, 93
performance dashboards, 86, 87
quality
checks, 84
control tools, 81
measurement, 88–90
RIE, 94
SIPOC
NVA, 82
NVA-R, 82
VA, 82
strive for perfection, 84
Toyota Production System, 81
training and skill acquisition, 92
value, 82
VBP, 88, 91
VSM, 83, 91, 93
Lexicon of Collaborative Care, 7
Likert-type scale, 182
Lower control limit (LCL), 85

M
Management competencies, 124
Marketing plan, 151
Medical ethics, 213
Medical psychology, 104
mHealth, 153
Multidisciplinary skills, 117
My Own Health Report (MOHR), 96

N
National Committee for Quality Assurance, 80
National Institute of Mental Health (NIMH), 22
Normal distribution curve, 192

O
Outlier, 190, 191

P
Patient-centered interventions, 77
Patient-centered medical home (PCMH), 20, 80, 124
Performance Improvement Model, 85
Plan-do-study-act (PDSA), 85, 93, 99–100
Population health management (PHM), 4, 5, 136
chronic illnesses, 69
components, 68
conceptual and operational shifts, 67
core competency skills, 71
cost-effective, 68, 72, 74
development planning guide, 73

effectiveness measures, 75
EHRs, 69
engagement, 77
history, 66
interprofessional team, 70
IPC, 66, 68
patient-centered interventions, 77
population identification, 76
and public health, 67, 68
reimbursement strategies, 70
risk stratification, 76
ROI, 74
SMART, 77
stakeholders, 69
team-based care, 71
workforce development, 76
Practice Integration Profile (PIP), vii, 7, 27
Practitioner performance evaluation, 54, 55, 58, 59
Preferred provider organization (PPO), 180
Primary care behavioral health (PCBH), 121–124, 133, 208
CFHA, 22
clinicians, 22
overview, 21
web-based training program, 24
Primary care physicians (PCP), 121
AHRQ, 17
antidepressant medications, 18, 19
biopsychosocial management, 21
IOM, 20
skill and comfort, 21
Pro forma, 129, 131
Pro forma approach, 122
Process and outcomes
care delivery, 6
5 Rs framework, 7
integrated care, 7
Professional decision-making tool, 217–219
Program evaluation
clinic, 178
health-care, 181
Public health, 67

Q
Quality improvement, 86–88, 94, 97, 98

R
Randomized controlled trial (RCT), 17–20, 185
Rapid Improvement Event (RIE), 94, 98, 99
RE-AIM model, 8
Research and evaluation paradigm, 7–8
Return on investment (ROI), 74
analysis, 136
calculation, 136
competencies, 130
costs, 120
Revenue
billing codes for reimbursement, 131
business case, 120
competencies, 128
Risk assessment, 151
Risk stratification, 76
Roles and responsibilities (RR), 107
Rubric
competency, 10
exposure, 9
skill acquisition, 10

S
Sales strategy, 152
Skewness
description, 191
normality assumptions, 197, 201
types, 193
Skill development, 37, 69
Stakeholders, 68, 69, 71
Statistical issues, 178, 179, 197
Statistical significance *vs* clinical significance, 195
Statistical test
decision tree, 186, 187
five-point Likert-type scale, 185
myriad statistical techniques, 186
Statistical training, 178
process-oriented approach, 179
Strategic planning, 151
Structure-process-outcomes model, 25
Study designs
biomedical research, 185, 186, 199
clustered data, 184
confounder, 182
statistical tests, 178, 181
Type I and Type II error, 183, 184
Substance Abuse and Mental Services Association and the Health Resources and Services Administration (SAMHSA-HRSA), 25
SWOT analysis, 156

T
Teaching approach, 71
Team-based care, 104

Team-based care (*cont.*)
  health education and clinical training, 104
  resources, 111–112
  training priorities, 110
Team-based education, 104
Team-based training, 105–109
Team performance, 105, 113–116
Teams and teamwork (TT), 109
Three worlds of healthcare service delivery, viii, 42–44, 49, 168
Training
  objectives and outcomes
    competency, 10–11
    exposure, 9
    levels, 8
    skill acquisition, 9–10
  workforce, 8
Training and development, 8
Training priorities, 114–116
Treat-to-target model, 23
Triple Aim, 4
  ACA (*see* Affordable Care Act (ACA))
  PHM, 4
  PIP, 7
Type I and Type II error
  hypothesis testing, 183, 184
  p-value, 183, 184

U
Upper control limit (UCL), 85

V
Value-based integrated behavioral health, 121
Value-based payment (VBP), 80, 121
Value-based reimbursement, 104
Values and ethics (VE), 106
Value stream map (VSM), 83, 88, 93, 96, 98

W
Workforce development, 41, 163
  evaluation, 51
  evaluation phase, 48
  IBH training, 23, 25
  implementation, 50
  implementation phase, 47, 48
  interconnected training phases, 49
  preparation, 50
  preparation phase, 47
Workforce development training
  CMEs, 211
  knowledge-based training, 210
  medical pathophysiology, 210
  reverse integration, 211
Workforce training, 103–105, 110, 215, 223

The manufacturer's authorised representative in the EU is Springer Nature Customer Service Centre GmbH, Europaplatz 3, 69115 Heidelberg, Germany. If you have any concerns regarding our products, please contact ProductSafety@springernature.com

Printed and bound by CPI Group (UK) Ltd, Croydon, CR0 4YY
30/09/2026
02225658-0005